Plant-Diet Manual

Healthy and tasty recipes to stay fit with taste

Carolyn J. Perez

This Book Included

Book 1:

THE PLANT-BASED DIET

Cook delicious and healthy Plant-Based recipes for weight loss.

Book 2:

PLANT-BASED DIET

Lose weight and get back in shape by following easy and delicious Plant-Based recipes.

Carolyn J. Perez

The Plant-Based Diet

Cook delicious and healthy Plant-Based recipes for weight loss

Carolyn J. Perez

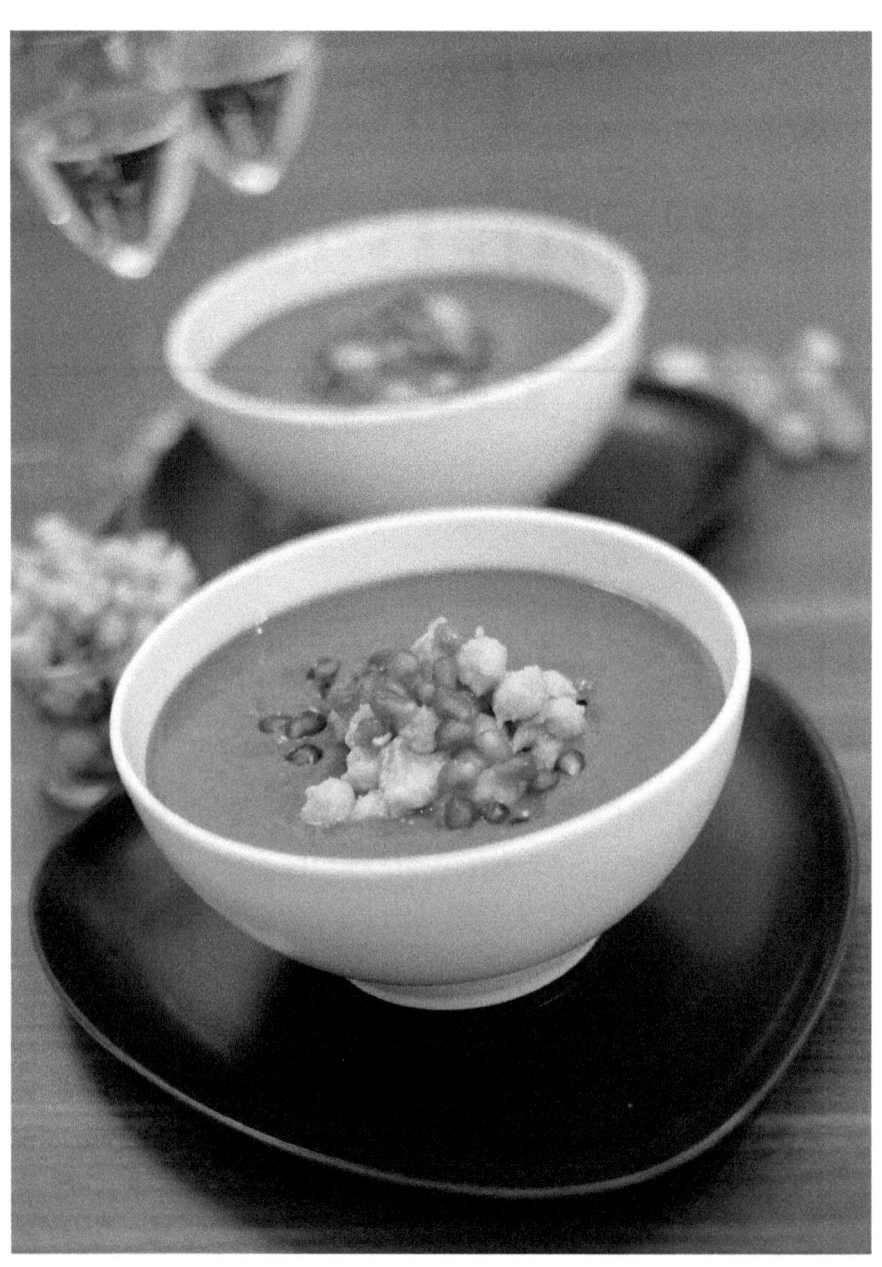

© **Copyright 2021 - All rights reserved.**

The content contained within this book may not be reproduced, duplicated or transmitted without direct written permission from the author or the publisher.

Under no circumstances will any blame or legal responsibility be held against the publisher, or author, for any damages, reparation, or monetary loss due to the information contained within this book. Either directly or indirectly.

Legal Notice:

This book is copyright protected. This book is only for personal use. You cannot amend, distribute, sell, use, quote or paraphrase any part, or the content within this book, without the consent of the author or publisher.

Disclaimer Notice:

Please note the information contained within this document is for educational and entertainment purposes only. All effort has been executed to present accurate, up to date, and reliable, complete information. No warranties of any kind are declared or implied. Readers acknowledge that the author is not engaging in the rendering of legal, financial, medical or professional advice. The content within this book has been derived from various sources. Please consult a licensed professional before attempting any techniques outlined in this book.

By reading this document, the reader agrees that under no circumstances is the author responsible for any losses, direct or indirect, which are incurred as a result of the use of information contained within this document, including, but not limited to, — errors, omissions, or inaccuracies.

Contents

INTRODUCTION 10
PLANT BASED DIET: WHAT ARE WE TALKING ABOUT? 12
MAIN DIFFERENCES BETWEEN VEGAN AND PLANT BASED DIET 14
    Chapter 1 Soup Recipes 24
    Bean soup, artichokes and peas 24
    Soup with potatoes, zucchinis and radishes 26
    Brown rice and fennel soup 28
    Broccoli soup and wholemeal spaghetti 30
    Cold soup of melon and green tomatoes 32
    Barley and tomato soup 34
    Minestrone with mixed vegetables 36
    Cream of lettuce 38
    Cream of celery 40
    Watermelon and tomato soup 42
    Carrot and beetroot soup 43
    Spelt soup and shallots 45
    Bean board soup 47
    Chickpeas with saffron 49
    Chickpea soup 51
    Cauliflower and chickpea soup 53
    Chickpea and shallot soup 56
    Cream of chickpeas 58
    Chickpea, spinach and potato soup 60
    Bean and potato soup 62
    Corn and bean soup 65
    Cold peas soup 67
CHAPTER 2 70
MAIN COURSES 70
    Nuggets of seitan with peppers 70
    Sandwich with flavoured tofu 72
    Amaranth and pumpkin croquettes 74
    Salad with tofu, pear and honey 77
    Cucumber, watermelon and mozzarella plant based salad 78
    Apple and fennel salad 79
    Mixed vegetable and fruit salad with chia seeds 80
    Greek salad with tofu 81

Chickpea and mushroom salad 82
Onion and walnut plum cake 83
Eggplant, tomatoes and plant based mozzarella 85
Baked seitan with capers, lemon and mint 86
Juniper and orange seitan 88
Seitan with herbs 89
Strips of tempeh with olives 90
Fried tofu with lemon 91
Ginger glazed tofu 93
Quiche with potatoes, zucchini and plant based mozzarella 95
Quiche with cherry tomatoes, vegan mozzarella and capers 97
Quiche with vegetables 98
Quiche with zucchini, zucchini flowers and plant based mozzarella 100
Potato, pumpkin and plant based mozzarella pie 102
Baked pumpkin, chickpeas and tofu 103
Roast seitan with apples 105
Green beans, potatoes and tofu 107
Vegetable cream buns 109
Tofu and almond meatballs 110

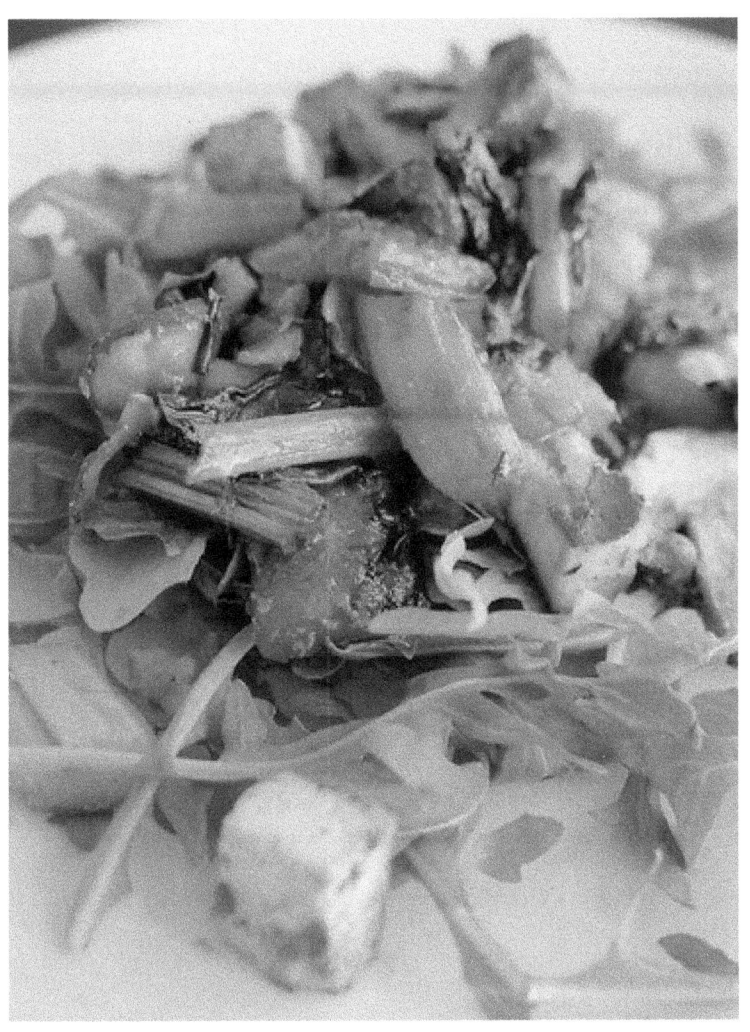

Introduction

It is a common thought to think that following a diet is necessarily linked to the concept of actual weight loss. However, this is not always the case: following a diet is often directly linked to the foods that we decide to include in our tables daily.

In addition, we do not always choose the best quality ingredients to cook our dishes.

Sometimes we are so rushed and unruly that we forget that we love our bodies. And what better cure than a healthy diet? Following a healthy diet should become more than an imposition or a punishment, but a real lifestyle.

Moreover, this is the Plant-based diet goal: not to impose a restrictive and sometimes impossible diet to follow, but to recreate a diet based on foods of natural origin and above all healthy. Therefore, the plant based represents a real food trend. However, as we will see it is much more than just a fashion trend, but a real lifestyle.

In addition, it is the aim of this text, or rather of this cookbook, to introduce you to the plant based discipline. And we will do it with a few theoretical explanations, just to make you understand what we are talking about and above all how to prepare it: there will be a purely practical part where you will find 50 recipes on the plant based. These recipes will be divided into appetizers, snacks, first and second courses, side dishes and finally a string of plant based desserts.

In the end, you will be spoiled for choice to start following this healthy dietary discipline.

Plant based diet: what are we talking about?

We already mentioned that more than a real weight loss diet the Plant based diet is a food discipline. Food discipline is enjoying great success not only because it is very fashionable, but because it applies such principles that can be perfectly integrated into our daily lives. The plant-based diet is a true approach to life, starting with nutrition: respect for one's health and body, first of all, which is reflected in respect for all forms of life and the planet in general.

As the word itself says, it deals with a food plan based, precisely on what comes from plants. However, simply calling it that way would be too simplistic.

It is a predominantly plant-based diet, but not only. It is not just about consuming vegetables but about taking natural foods: not industrially processed, not treated, and not deriving from the exploitation of resources and animals, preferably zero km.

So it could be a discipline that aims not only at environmental saving but also at the economic one: think about what advantages, in fact, at the level of your pockets you can have if you apply the principle of 0Km and therefore to be able to harvest your vegetables directly from your garden.

Environmental savings do not only mean pollution reduction: the ethical component (present exclusively in the vegan diet, for example) is combined with a strong will to health. This means that the plant based, in addition to not preferring foods that exploit animals, is also based on foods that are especially unprocessed, fresh, healthy, balanced, light, and rich in essential nutrients. In practice, it is a plant-based diet but not vegan / vegetarian, emphasizing the quality and wholesomeness of foods rather than on their moral value, albeit with great attention to sustainability. Such a lifestyle could therefore be of help, not only to our health, but also to create a more sustainable world for future generations.

Main differences between Vegan and Plant based diet

The plant-based diet is often associated with the vegan diet. This is because both plan to include cruelty free foods that do not involve any animal exploitation.

Furthermore, they are associated precisely because they are both predominantly plant-based.

However, there are some pretty obvious differences between these two diets.

First of all, precisely for the reasoning behind the prevalence of plants.

It is well known that even the vegan diet provides a diet based on foods of plant origin: unlike the plant-based diet, however, nothing of animal derivation is allowed, neither direct nor indirect, nor other products - clothing or accessories - which include the exploitation of animals.

No eggs, no milk, no honey, no leather, so to speak, and not only: in its most rigorous meanings, veganism does not even include the use of yeasts, as the bacteria that compose them are indisputably living beings.

A vegan diet can be balanced if the person who leads it knows well the foods and their combinations, the necessary supplements, and their body's reaction to the lack of certain foods.

On the contrary, the Plant-Based diet is on the one hand more relaxed, on the other more stringent.

What does it mean?

This means that it is on the one hand more relaxed because it is plant-based, but not exclusively vegetable: products of animal origin are allowed, in moderate quantities, but under only one condition, namely the excellent quality of the food itself and its certified origin. For example, eggs can be consumed occasionally but only if very fresh, possibly at zero km, from free-range farms where the hens are not exploited but can live outdoors without constraints.

It is also a somewhat more stringent philosophy than veganism precisely for this reason: as long as it is 100% vegetable, the vegan also consumes heavily processed foods, such as industrial fries. Therefore, the vegan can also eat junk foods or snacks. Conversely, plant-based dieters would never admit highly refined foods of this type.

Both dietary approaches are conscious and do not involve the consumption of meat. However, if vegans are driven by ethical reasons, those who follow a plant-based diet also reject everything processed on an industrial level and unhealthy.

A plant-based diet is a diet that aims to eliminate industrially processed foods and, therefore, potentially more harmful to health. It is based on the consumption of fruit and vegetables, whole grains and avoiding (or minimizing) animal products and processed foods. This means that vegan desserts made with refined sugar or bleached flour are also covered.

There is also a substantial difference between the philosophies behind the two diets. As we said in the previous paragraph and above, the ethical component, which is based on the refusal of any food of animal origin, plays a lot in veganism. While for the plant based is not a purely moral and moralistic discourse but on the real thought of being able to keep healthy with the food discipline and be respectful of the environment surrounding us.

Plant based diet full shopping list. What to eat and what to avoid

Now we can examine the complete shopping list of the plant based diet.
Let's briefly summarize the principles on which this particular type of diet is based:

- Emphasizes whole, minimally processed foods.
- Limits or avoids animal products.
- Focuses on plants, including vegetables, fruits, whole grains, legumes, seeds and nuts, which should make up most of what you eat.
- Excludes refined foods, like added sugars, white flour and processed oils.
- Pays special attention to food quality, promoting locally sourced, organic food whenever possible.

As for what you can usually eat, we can say the general consumption of:

- Wholegrain and flours
- extra virgin olive oil

- Seasonal fruit and vegetables: these foods are the basis of every meal.
- In this diet you can also eat sweets but only and exclusively homemade and with controlled raw materials, simple and not very refined, preferably of vegetable origin - for example by replacing milk with soy or rice drinks, and eggs with other natural thickeners such as flaxseed, or simple ripe banana.
- You can also consume nuts and seeds.

As for absolutely forbidden foods, there are all those ready-made and processed:

- ready-made sauces
- chips
- biscuits
- various kinds of snacks
- sugary cereals,
- Spreads, snacks and many other notoriously unhealthy foods.
- Junk food and fast food are therefore absolutely banned
- Sugar beverages

Regarding the complete shopping list:
- Fruits: Berries, citrus fruits, pears, peaches, pineapple, bananas, etc.
- Vegetables: Kale, spinach, tomatoes, broccoli, cauliflower, carrots, asparagus, peppers, etc.
- Starchy vegetables: Potatoes, sweet potatoes, butternut squash, etc.
- Whole grains: Brown rice, rolled oats, spelt, quinoa, brown rice pasta, barley, etc.
- Healthy fats with omega 3: Avocados, olive oil, coconut oil, unsweetened coconut, etc.
- Legumes: Peas, chickpeas, lentils, peanuts, beans, black beans, etc.
- Seeds, nuts and nut butter: Almonds, cashews, macadamia nuts, pumpkin seeds, sunflower seeds, natural peanut butter, tahini, etc.
- Unsweetened plant-based milk: Coconut milk, almond milk, cashew milk, etc.
- Spices, herbs and seasonings: Basil, rosemary, turmeric, curry, black pepper, salt, etc.
- Condiments: Salsa, mustard, nutritional yeast, soy sauce, vinegar, lemon juice, etc.

- Plant-based protein: Tofu, tempeh, seitan, and plant based protein sources or powders with no added sugar or artificial ingredients.
- Beverages: Coffee, tea, sparkling water, etc.

There is the chance to add food of animal origin very rarely, for example if you have specific nutritional needs or if it has been strongly recommended by your doctor. Anyway, if supplementing your plant-based diet with animal products choose quality products from grocery stores or, better yet, purchase them from local farms.

- Eggs: Pasture-raised when possible.
- Poultry: Free-range, organic when possible.
- Beef and pork: Pastured or grass-fed when possible.
- Seafood: Wild-caught from sustainable fisheries when possible.
- Dairy: Organic dairy products from pasture-raised animals whenever possible.

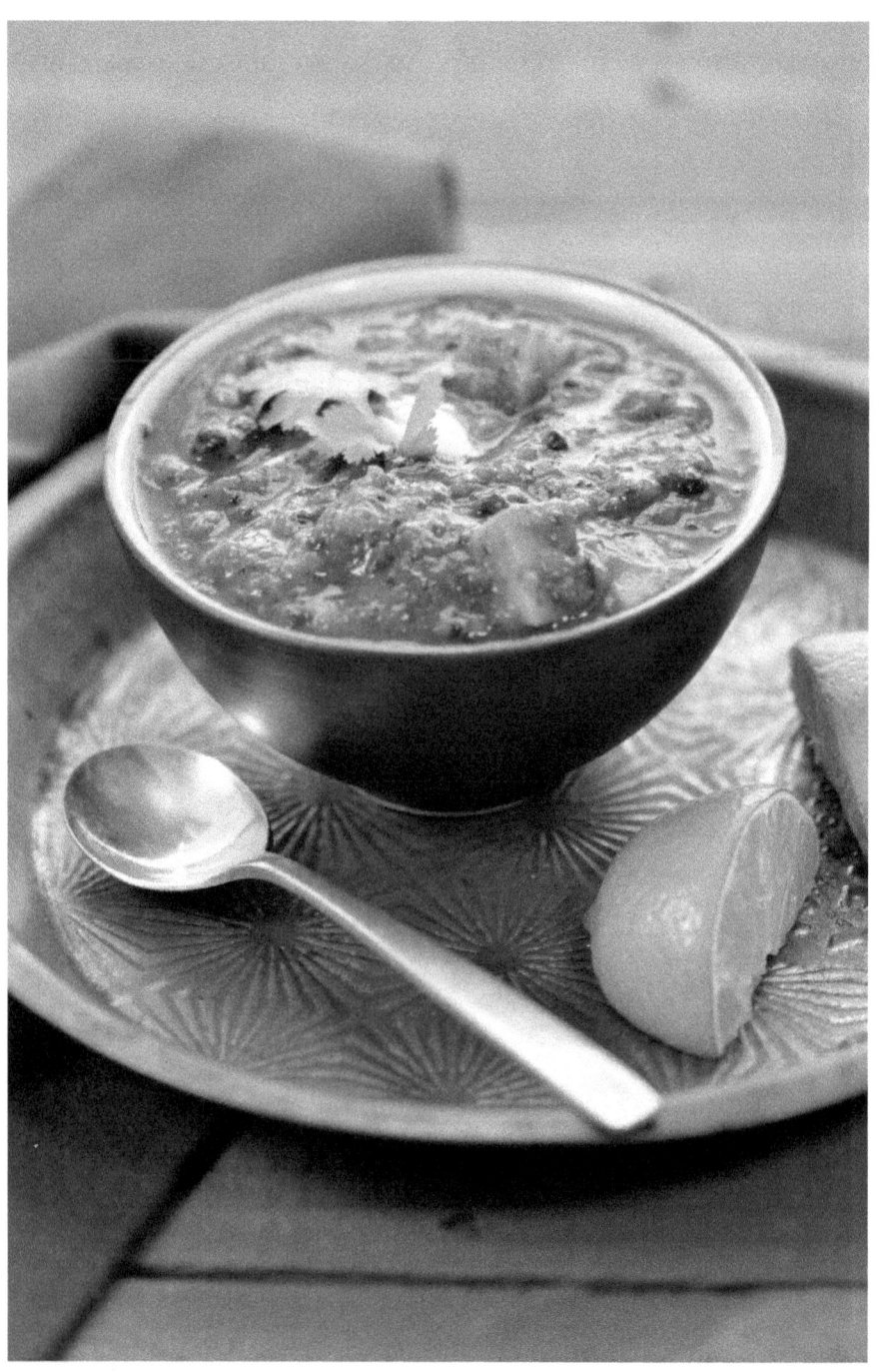

Chapter 1 Soup Recipes

Bean soup, artichokes and peas

PREPARATION TIME: 20 minutes
COOKING TIME: 20 minutes

CALORIES: 310

INGREDIENTS FOR 4 SERVINGS
- 200 grams of broad beans
- 200 grams of peas
- 4 artichokes
- One lemon
- 2 shallots
- 2 cloves of garlic
- A sprig of chopped parsley
- 800 ml of hot vegetable broth
- Olive oil to taste
- Salt and Pepper to taste

DIRECTIONS
1. Start with the artichokes, remove the stalk and hard leaves, divide them in half, and remove the internal beard. Cut them into wedges and put them in a bowl with water and lemon juice.

2. Wash the broad beans and peas under running water and then let them drain.
3. Peel and wash the shallots and garlic cloves and then chop them.
4. Put two tablespoons of oil in a saucepan to heat. Now put the shallots and garlic to brown for a couple of minutes.
5. Put the drained artichokes and sauté them for 3 minutes.
6. Now add the broad beans and peas. Season with salt and pepper, stir and cook for a couple of minutes.
7. Now add the broth and cook for 20 minutes.
8. When the vegetables are well cooked, turn off and put the soup on serving plates.

Soup with potatoes, zucchinis and radishes

PREPARATION TIME: 20 minutes
COOKING TIME: 25 minutes

CALORIES: 145

INGREDIENTS FOR 4 SERVINGS
- 2 potatoes
- 1 shallot
- 2 radishes
- 500 grams of zucchinis
- Olive oil to taste
- Salt and pepper to taste

DIRECTIONS
1. Peel the shallot, wash it and chop it.
2. Peel the potatoes, wash them thoroughly and then cut them into cubes.
3. Wash the zucchinis and then cut them into slices.
4. Wash the radishes and cut them into thin slices.
5. Heat a drizzle of oil in a saucepan and then put the shallot to brown.
6. Add the potatoes, season with salt and pepper, mix and then add half a glass of water.
7. Cook for 15 minutes and then add the zucchinis.

8. Cook for another 10 minutes.
9. After cooking time turn off and blend everything with an immersion blender.
10. Now put the soup on the plates, decorate with radishes, season with a drizzle of oil and serve.

Brown rice and fennel soup

PREPARATION TIME: 5 minutes

COOKING TIME: 35 minutes
CALORIES: 437

INGREDIENTS FOR 4 SERVINGS

- 280 grams of brown rice
- 600 grams of fennel
- 1 onion
- 1 sprig of chopped parsley
- 1 litre of vegetable broth
- 1 sachet of saffron
- Olive oil to taste
- Salt and pepper to taste

DIRECTIONS
1. Remove the tough outer leaves and the beard from the fennel and then wash them under running water. Cut them, first in half and then into thin slices.
2. Peel and wash the onion and then chop it.
3. Heat a tablespoon of oil in a saucepan. Put the chopped onion and brown it for 2 minutes, stirring often.
4. Add the fennel, stir and cook with the pan covered with a lid.

5. Add the rice and sauté for 2 minutes.
6. Add the vegetable broth and cook until the rice is cooked al dente.
7. Add the saffron and mix well to fully incorporate it with the other ingredients.
8. Now you can turn off, put the soup on the serving plates and serve.

Broccoli soup and wholemeal spaghetti

PREPARATION TIME: 20 minutes

COOKING TIME: 40 minutes
CALORIES: 200

INGREDIENTS FOR 4 SERVINGS
- 800 grams of broccoli flowers
- 300 grams of potatoes
- 80 grams of wholemeal spaghetti
- 1 clove of garlic
- 1 litre of vegetable broth
- Olive oil to taste
- Salt and pepper to taste

DIRECTIONS
1. Start by preparing the garlic oil.
2. Peel and wash the garlic and then chop it. Put it in a small bowl covered with olive oil. Keep aside until the soup is ready.
3. Peel the potatoes, wash them and then cut them into cubes.
4. Wash and let the broccoli flowers drain.
5. Heat two tablespoons of oil in a saucepan and as soon as it is hot, brown the potatoes and broccoli flowers.

6. Mix well, season with salt and pepper and then add the broth.
7. Cook for 20 minutes.
8. After 20 minutes, lower the heat and blend everything with an immersion blender.
9. Break up the spaghetti and add them to the soup. Stir and continue cooking for another 10 minutes.
10. Now turn off and put the soup on serving plates. Season with garlic oil, a little pepper and serve.

Cold soup of melon and green tomatoes

PREPARATION TIME: 15 minutes+30 minutes to rest in fridge
CALORIES: 215

INGREDIENTS FOR 4 SERVINGS
- 2 melons
- 2 green tomatoes
- A tablespoon of chopped chives
- Olive oil to taste
- Salt and Pepper to taste
- 1 teaspoon of paprika

DIRECTIONS
1. Peel the melon, remove the seeds, wash the pulp and then cut it into cubes.
2. Put the melon pulp in the glass of the blender together with salt, pepper, paprika and chives.
3. Blend at high speed until you get a smooth and homogeneous mixture.
4. Put the mixture in a bowl and put it to rest in the fridge for 30 minutes.
5. Meanwhile, wash the tomatoes, cut them in half and remove the pulp and seeds. Cut the rest of the tomatoes

into cubes.
6. Now take the soup from the fridge and divide it into serving plates.
7. Sprinkle with tomatoes, drizzle with a drizzle of oil and serve.

Barley and tomato soup

PREPARATION TIME: 25 minutes

COOKING TIME: 40 minutes
CALORIES: 240

INGREDIENTS FOR 4 SERVINGS
- 150 grams of green beans
- 50 grams of pearl barley
- 100 grams of tomato pulp
- 1 potato
- 1 shallot
- 1 tablespoon of thyme leaves
- 2.5 litres of hot vegetable broth
- Olive oil to taste
- Salt and pepper to taste

DIRECTIONS
1. Start with the barley. Put it in a bowl and cover it with cold water, let it soak for 15 minutes. After 15 minutes, drain and set aside.
2. Check the green beans, wash them and cut them into small pieces.
3. Peel the potato, wash it and cut it into cubes.
4. Peel and wash the shallot and then chop it.

5. Heat two tablespoons of oil in a saucepan.
6. Brown the shallot for 1 minute.
7. Put the tomato pulp, season with salt and pepper and mix.
8. After 5 minutes, add the broth, potato and barley.
9. Cook for 20 minutes and then add the green beans.
10. Continue cooking for another 20 minutes and over medium heat.
11. After 20 minutes, season with salt and pepper, mix and turn off.
12. Put the soup on plates, season with oil and pepper, sprinkle with thyme flowers and serve.

Minestrone with mixed vegetables

PREPARATION TIME: 20 minutes
COOKING TIME: 30 minutes
CALORIES: 210

INGREDIENTS FOR 4 SERVINGS
- 1 carrot
- 1 potato
- 1 onion
- 1 leek
- 250 grams of broccoli flowers
- 1 tomato
- 2 sprigs of parsley
- 2 litres of vegetable broth
- Olive oil to taste
- Salt and pepper to taste

DIRECTIONS
1. Wash and dry the parsley and then chop it.
2. Peel and wash the carrot and then cut it into cubes.
3. Peel and wash the potato and then cut it into cubes.
4. Peel the onion and leek, wash them and then cut them into thin slices.
5. Wash the broccoli flowers and then let them drain.

6. Wash the tomato and then cut it into cubes.
7. Put two tablespoons of oil in a pan and as soon as it is hot, put the leek and onion to fry for a couple of minutes.
8. Add the potato, carrot, and mix.
9. Season with salt and pepper and then add the broth.
10. Cook for 10 minutes and then add the broccoli and tomato.
11. Continue cooking for another 20 minutes, stirring occasionally.
12. As soon as the minestrone is cooked, turn it off and put it on serving plates.
13. Drizzle with a drizzle of oil and serve.

Cream of lettuce

PREPARATION TIME: 15 minutes
COOKING TIME: 25 minutes
CALORIES: 80

INGREDIENTS FOR 4 SERVINGS
- 500 grams of lettuce
- 15 grams of wholemeal breadcrumbs
- 2 shallots
- 1 teaspoon of paprika
- 350 ml of vegetable broth
- Olive oil to taste
- Salt and pepper to taste

DIRECTIONS
1. Peel the shallots, wash them and then cut them into slices.
2. Wash the lettuce leaves one by one, and then dry them. Cut them into small pieces.
3. Heat two tablespoons of olive oil in a saucepan and as soon as it is hot, put the shallots to dry.
4. Now add the lettuce, mix well and sauté for a minute.
5. Season with salt and pepper, mix and add the vegetable broth.

6. Cook for 20 minutes.
7. After 20 minutes, lower the heat and blend everything with an immersion blender.
8. Now add the breadcrumbs and cook another 5 minutes, the time necessary to thicken the cream.
9. Now turn off and put on plates. Season with oil and a little pepper and serve.

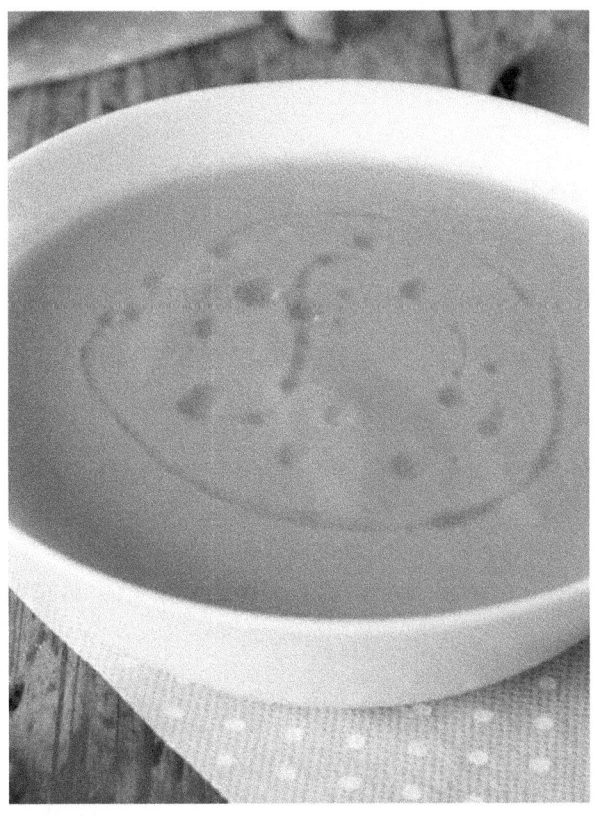

Cream of celery

PREPARATION TIME: 20 minutes
COOKING TIME: 25 minutes
CALORIES: 172

INGREDIENTS FOR 4 SERVINGS
- 1 kilo of celery
- 500 grams of potatoes
- Half onion
- Olive oil to taste
- Salt and pepper to taste

DIRECTIONS
1. Peel and wash the onion and then chop it.
2. Remove the celery bases and side filaments, then wash them and cut them into small pieces, including the leaves.
3. Peel the potatoes, wash them and then cut them into cubes.
4. Heat a tablespoon of oil in a saucepan and as soon as it is hot, put the onion to fry.
5. Now add the potatoes and cook for 5 minutes.
6. Now add the celery, season with salt and pepper.
7. Stir and add 1.5 litres of water.

8. Cook for 20 minutes and then turn off.
9. With an immersion blender until you, get a velvety and homogeneous cream.
10. Put the soup on plates, season with oil and serve.

Watermelon and tomato soup

PREPARATION TIME: 20 minutes
CALORIES: 70

INGREDIENTS FOR 4 SERVINGS
- 400 grams of watermelon
- 2 tomatoes
- 1 sprig of parsley
- 4 basil leaves
- Olive oil to taste
- Salt and pepper to taste

DIRECTIONS
1. Peel the watermelon and remove all the seeds. Now cut it into cubes.
2. Wash the tomatoes and then cut them into cubes.
3. Wash and dry the parsley and basil.
4. Put all the ingredients in a bowl.
5. Take an immersion blender and blend until you get a smooth and homogeneous cream.
6. Put the soup on the plates, season with oil, salt and pepper and serve.

Carrot and beetroot soup

PREPARATION TIME: 20 minutes
COOKING TIME: 65 minutes

CALORIES: 190

INGREDIENTS FOR 4 SERVINGS
- 300 grams of beets
- 1 jar of soy yogurt
- 40 grams of oat flour
- 30 grams of soy butter
- 1.5 litres of vegetable broth
- 2 carrots
- 1 shallot
- 1 tablespoon of apple cider vinegar
- Salt and pepper to taste

DIRECTIONS
1. Peel and wash the shallot and then chop it.
2. Peel and wash the carrot and then cut it into cubes.
3. Peel the beetroot, wash it and cut it with cubes.
4. Put the butter to melt in a pan and as soon as it melts, put the flour to toast.
5. Stir constantly until you get a smooth, lump-free cream.
6. Now add the carrots, beets and shallots.

7. Stir, season with salt, pepper, and cook for 5 minutes.
8. Now add the vegetable broth.
9. Cook for 60 minutes.
10. After 60 minutes, turn off and blend everything with an immersion blender.
11. Now add the yogurt and mix until it is completely blended with the soup.
12. Now put the soup on the plates, season it with oil and pepper and serve.

Spelt soup and shallots

PREPARATION TIME: 20 minutes

COOKING TIME: 55 minutes
CALORIES: 366

INGREDIENTS FOR 4 SERVINGS
- 300 grams of spelt
- 2 shallots
- 1.5 litres of vegetable broth
- 2 tablespoons of tomato puree
- 1 teaspoon of thyme leaves
- Olive oil to taste
- Salt and pepper to taste

DIRECTIONS
1. Peel and wash the shallots and then cut them into thin slices.
2. Rinse the spelled and let it drain.
3. Heat two tablespoons of oil in a saucepan.
4. As soon as the oil is hot, put the shallots to brown.
5. Cook for 2-3 minutes and then add the spelt.
6. Stir, cook for a few minutes and then add the broth, tomato sauce, salt and pepper.
7. Bring to a boil and then continue cooking for another 40

minutes.
8. Check the cooking before turning off and if the spelled is not cooked yet, continue for another 5 minutes.
9. When cooked, turn off and put the soup on the plates.
10. Season with thyme and pepper flowers and serve.

Bean board soup

PREPARATION TIME: 20 minutes
COOKING TIME: 35 minutes
CALORIES: 183

INGREDIENTS FOR 4 SERVINGS
- 1 kilo of broad beans already peeled
- 1 shallot
- Olive oil to taste
- 1 tablespoon of thyme leaves
- Salt and pepper to taste

DIRECTIONS
1. Peel the shallot and then chop it.
2. Wash the broad beans and then let them drain.
3. Heat a tablespoon of olive oil in a saucepan and then brown the shallot.
4. Sauté for a couple of minutes and then add the beans.
5. Stir, season with salt, pepper, and sauté for 5 minutes, stirring often.
6. Now add 1.5 litres of hot water and cook for 30 minutes.
7. After 30 minutes, take a ladle of broad beans and place them in the glass of a blender.

8. Blend until you get a smooth and homogeneous cream.
9. Return the cream obtained to the pan with the other beans and mix.
10. Put the soup on the plates, season with oil and pepper, sprinkle with the thyme flowers and serve.

Chickpeas with saffron

PREPARATION TIME: 10 minutes
COOKING TIME: 2 hours and 15 minutes

CALORIES: 327

INGREDIENTS FOR 4 SERVINGS
- 300 grams of chickpeas
- 200 grams of tomato pulp
- 1 shallot
- 1 sachet of saffron
- 2 bay leaves
- Olive oil to taste
- Salt and pepper

DIRECTIONS
1. Start by preparing the chickpeas. Put them in a pot with plenty of water and salt.
2. Add the bay leaves that you have previously washed.
3. Cook the chickpeas and bay leaves for about 2 hours.
4. When they are ready, remove the bay leaf, drain the chickpeas and set aside the cooking liquid.
5. Peel and wash the shallot and then chop it.
6. Heat a little oil in a pan and as soon as it is hot, brown the shallot.

7. As soon as it is golden, add the tomato pulp.
8. Season with salt and pepper, stir and cook for 5 minutes.
9. Take 100 ml of the cooking liquid from the chickpeas and put the saffron to melt.
10. Now put the liquid with the saffron in the pan with the tomatoes.
11. Mix and add the chickpeas. Cook for another 5 minutes, adjust if necessary with salt, pepper, and turn off.
12. Put the chickpeas on plates and serve.

Chickpea soup

PREPARATION TIME: 35 minutes
COOKING TIME: 2 hours

CALORIES: 329

INGREDIENTS FOR 4 SERVINGS
- 300 grams of chickpeas
- 2 carrots
- 1 shallot
- 4 sage leaves
- Olive oil to taste
- Salt and pepper to taste

DIRECTIONS
1. Soak the chickpeas in a bowl with water and baking soda the night before cooking them.
2. When they are ready to be cooked, drain them, rinse them under running water and let them drain.
3. Peel and wash the shallot and chop it.
4. Wash and dry the sage leaves.
5. Peel and wash the carrots and then chop them.
6. Put a little oil to heat in a pot and then fry the shallot and carrots for a couple of minutes.
7. Now add the sage leaves and mix.

8. Add the chickpeas, season with salt and pepper and cover with hot water.
9. Bring to a boil, then cover with a lid, leaving a small crack, and cook for 2 hours.
10. When the soup is ready, put it on plates, season with a drizzle of oil and serve.

Cauliflower and chickpea soup

PREPARATION TIME: 20 minutes
COOKING TIME: 30 minutes

INGREDIENTS FOR 4 SERVINGS
- 1 cauliflower
- 250 grams of cooked chickpeas
- 400 ml of coconut milk
- 1 tablespoon of turmeric
- 1 clove of garlic
- 20 grams of grated ginger
- 400 ml of vegetable broth
- Olive oil to taste
- Salt and pepper to taste

DIRECTIONS
1. Peel and wash the garlic and then chop it.
2. Remove the stalk from the cauliflowers and keep only the flowers, wash them and let them drain.
3. Put a tablespoon of oil in a saucepan and as soon as it is hot, put the garlic to brown for a couple of minutes.
4. Add the turmeric and ginger, stir and cook for another 2 minutes.
5. Now add the coconut milk and bring to a boil.

6. Now add the cauliflower flowers and cook for about twenty minutes.
7. Now add the chickpeas and cook for another 5 minutes.
8. Season with salt and pepper, stir and then turn off.
9. Transfer the soup to serving dishes, season with oil and serve.

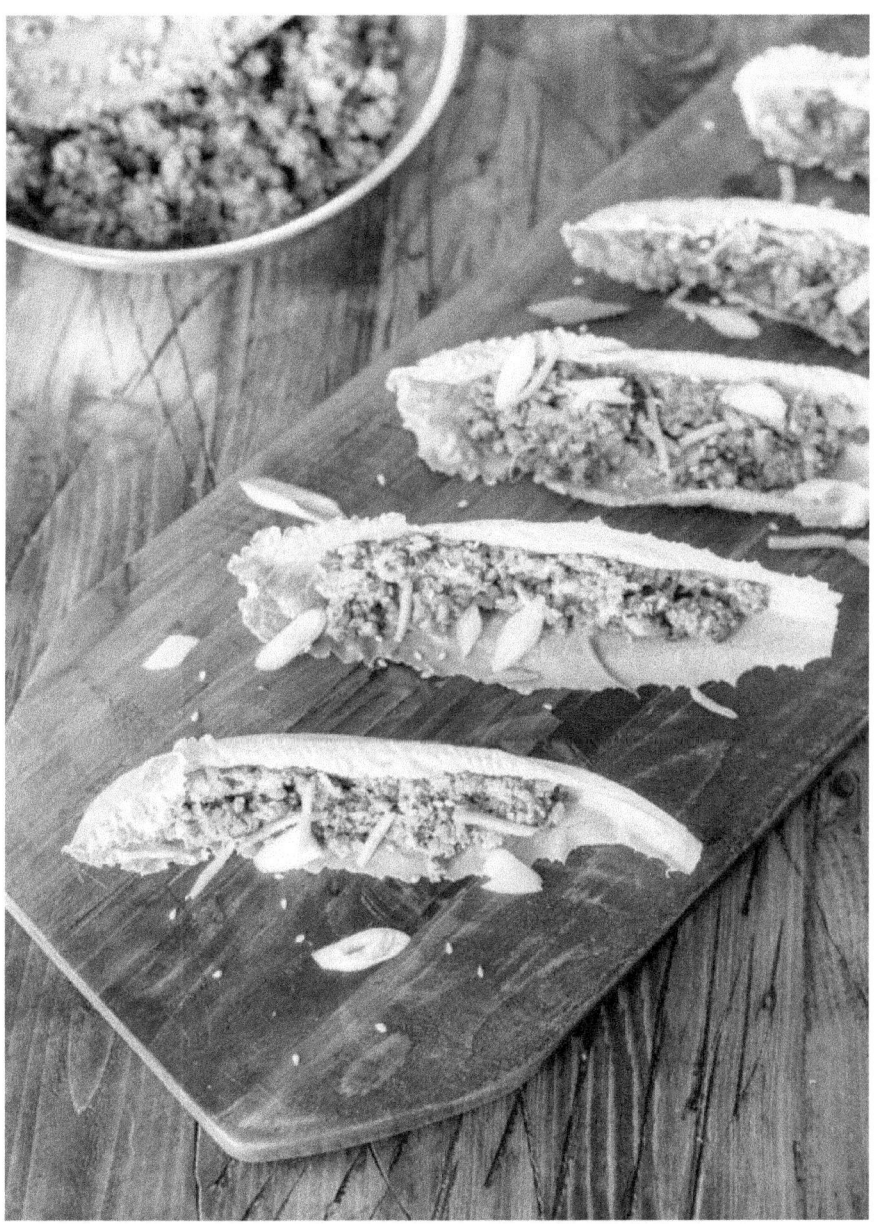

Chickpea and shallot soup

PREPARATION TIME: 15 minutes

COOKING TIME: 60 minutes
CALORIES: 531

INGREDIENTS FOR 4 SERVINGS
- 500 grams of cooked chickpeas
- 2 shallots
- 1 carrot
- 2 slices of cereal bread
- 500 ml of vegetal broth
- Olive oil to taste
- Salt and pepper to taste

DIRECTIONS
1. Peel and wash the carrot and then chop it.
2. Peel and wash the shallots and then cut them into slices.
3. Put a tablespoon of olive oil in a pan, and when it is hot, put the carrot and shallots to brown.
4. Add the chickpeas. Season with salt and pepper and let them brown for a couple of minutes.
5. Cover the chickpeas with the vegetable broth and bring to a boil.

6. Cook for about an hour and if necessary add more broth or hot water.
7. In the meantime, cut the bread into cubes and put it in a pan.
8. Toast it and when it is crunchy on the outside, turn off.
9. Peel and wash the carrot and then chop it.
10. Peel and wash the shallots and then cut them into slices.
11. Put a tablespoon of olive oil in a pan, and when it is hot, put the carrot and shallots to brown.
12. Add the chickpeas. Season with salt and pepper and let them brown for a couple of minutes.
13. Cover the chickpeas with the vegetable broth and bring to a boil.
14. Cook for about an hour and if necessary add more broth or hot water.
15. In the meantime, cut the bread into cubes and put it in a pan.
16. Toast it and when it is crunchy on the outside, turn off.
17. As soon as the soup is cooked, transfer it to serving plates. Season with a drizzle of oil, place the croutons and serve.

Cream of chickpeas

PREPARATION TIME: 5 minutes
COOKING TIME: 25 minutes

CALORIES: 250

INGREDIENTS FOR 4 SERVINGS
- 200 grams of already boiled chickpeas
- 1 shallot
- 1 carrot
- 2 cloves of garlic
- 1 litre of vegetable broth
- 1 tablespoon of sesame seeds
- Olive oil to taste
- Salt and pepper to taste.

DIRECTIONS
1. Peel and wash the shallot, the garlic cloves and the carrot and then chop them.
2. Heat a tablespoon of oil in a saucepan and then add garlic, carrot and shallot to fry.
3. Now add the chickpeas and vegetable broth and cook for about 20 minutes.
4. After 20 minutes, season with salt and pepper, mix and turn off.

5. With an immersion blender, blend everything until you get a smooth and homogeneous mixture.
6. Put the cream in serving dishes, season with oil, sprinkle with sesame seeds and serve.

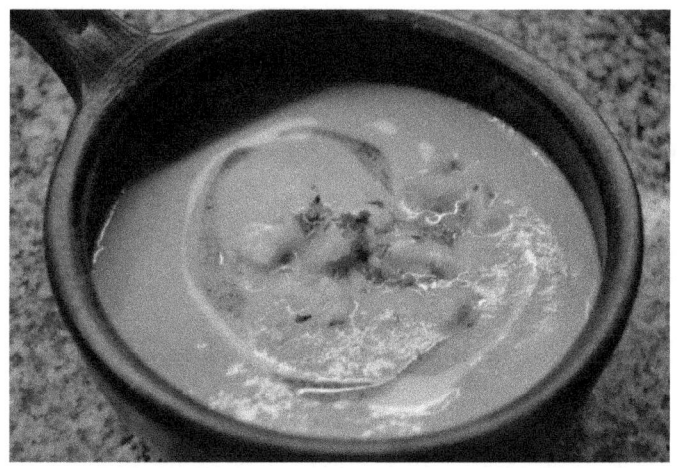

Chickpea, spinach and potato soup

PREPARATION TIME: 25 minutes
COOKING TIME: 30 minutes

CALORIES: 257

INGREDIENTS FOR 4 SERVINGS
- 400 grams of cooked chickpeas
- 2 potatoes
- 100 grams of spinach
- 2 tomatoes
- 100 ml of vegetable broth
- 1 clove of garlic
- Olive oil to taste
- Salt and pepper to taste

DIRECTIONS
1. Peel and wash the garlic and then chop it.
2. Peel the potatoes, wash them thoroughly and then cut them into cubes.
3. Wash the tomatoes and then cut them into cubes.
4. Heat a tablespoon of oil in a pan and then put the garlic to brown for a couple of minutes.
5. Now add the potatoes, mix and sauté them for 5 minutes.

6. Add the tomatoes, stir and after a couple of minutes add the chickpeas.
7. Season with salt and pepper, stir and add the broth. Cook for 20 minutes.
8. In the meantime, wash and dry the spinach.
9. Add them to the chickpeas, potatoes, and cook for another 5 minutes.
10. When the vegetables are well cooked, turn off.
11. Put the soup on plates, season with olive oil and serve.

Bean and potato soup

PREPARATION TIME: 30 minutes
COOKING TIME: 2 hours and 30 minutes

CALORIES: 526

INGREDIENTS FOR 4 SERVINGS
- 500 grams of beans
- 150 grams of potatoes
- 2 carrots
- 1 shallot
- 3 cloves of garlic
- 3 tablespoons of tomato sauce
- 2 sprigs of rosemary
- Vegetable broth to taste
- Olive oil to taste
- Salt and pepper to taste

DIRECTIONS
1. Start the preparation the night before, leaving the beans to soak in cold water overnight.
2. Now take the beans, drain them, put them in a pot with water and salt, and bring to a boil. Cook them for about an hour from the beginning of the boil.
3. In the meantime, peel and wash the shallot and then

chop it.
4. Peel and wash the carrots and then chop them.
5. Peel the potatoes, wash them thoroughly and then cut them into slices.
6. Heat a little oil in a pan and when it is hot, brown the shallot for a couple of minutes.
7. Add the carrot and continue for another minute.
8. Now put the potatoes. Season with salt and pepper and then add the vegetable broth until they are completely covered.
9. Cook until the potatoes are soft.
10. Now add the tomato puree, stir and cook for another 2 minutes.
11. Now put the potatoes in the pot with the beans. Mix and cook for an hour.
12. Meanwhile wash the rosemary.
13. Peel and wash the garlic cloves.
14. Put 4 tablespoons of oil in a pan and when hot, add the garlic and rosemary.
15. Cook for a couple of minutes and then put it in a bowl.
16. As soon as the soup is ready, divide it into plates, season with the garlic and rosemary flavoured oil and serve.

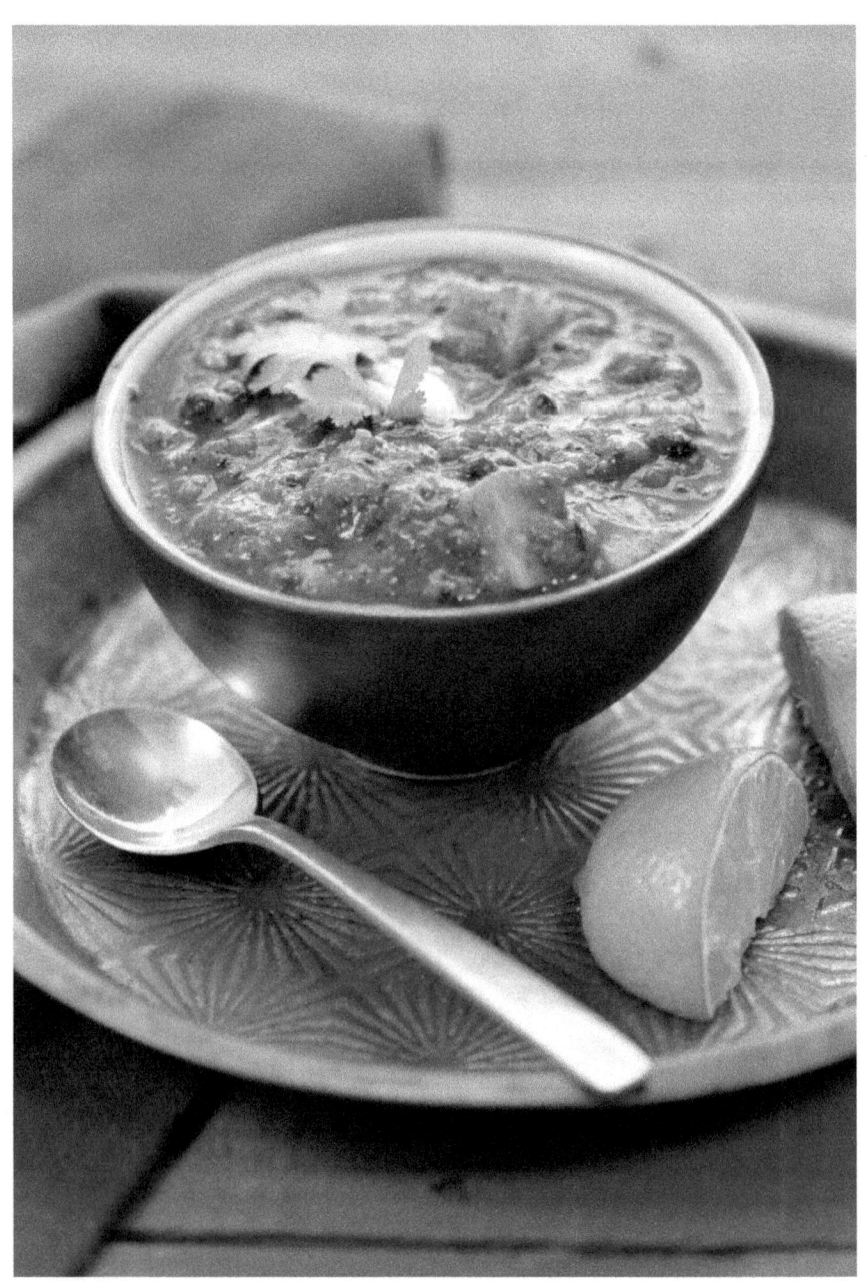

17.

Corn and bean soup

PREPARATION TIME: 10

COOKING TIME: 46
CALORIES: 506

INGREDIENTS FOR 4 SERVINGS
- 300 grams of beans
- 400 grams of corn kernels
- 2 potatoes
- 2 tomatoes
- 1 clove of garlic
- 750 ml of vegetable broth
- olive oil to taste
- salt and pepper to taste

DIRECTIONS
1. Peel, wash and chop the garlic.
2. Put a little oil in a saucepan and brown the garlic for a couple of minutes.
3. Now pour the vegetable broth and cook for 40 minutes.
4. In the meantime, peel the potatoes, wash them and then

cut them into cubes.
5. Wash the tomatoes and then cut them into cubes.
6. Heat the oil in another pan and as soon as it is hot, brown the corn, potatoes and tomatoes for 5 minutes.
7. Season with salt and pepper, mix and add 600 ml of water.
8. Cook for 30 minutes.
9. After 30 minutes, drain the vegetables and put them in the pot with the beans.
10. Mix well and cook for another 5 minutes.
11. Turn off, put in serving dishes, season with a little oil and serve.

Cold peas soup

PREPARATION TIME: 15 minutes+15 minutes to rest in fridge

COOKING TIME: 10 minutes
CALORIES: 147

INGREDIENTS FOR 4 SERVINGS
- 500 grams of peas
- 400 ml of vegetable broth
- 2 tablespoons of soymilk cream
- Salt and pepper to taste
- Olive oil to taste
- 4 mint leaves

DIRECTIONS
1. Wash the peas and let them drain.
2. Bring a pot of water and salt to a boil and then cook the peas for 10 minutes.
3. In the meantime, wash and dry the mint leaves.
4. Drain them, pass them under cold water and then put them in the glass of the blender. Add the vegetable broth and blend for a minute.
5. Add the soymilk cream, salt, mint and pepper and blend again.
6. Put the blender glass to rest in the fridge for 15 minutes.

7. After 15 minutes, take the soup, put it on serving plates, season with a drizzle of oil and serve.

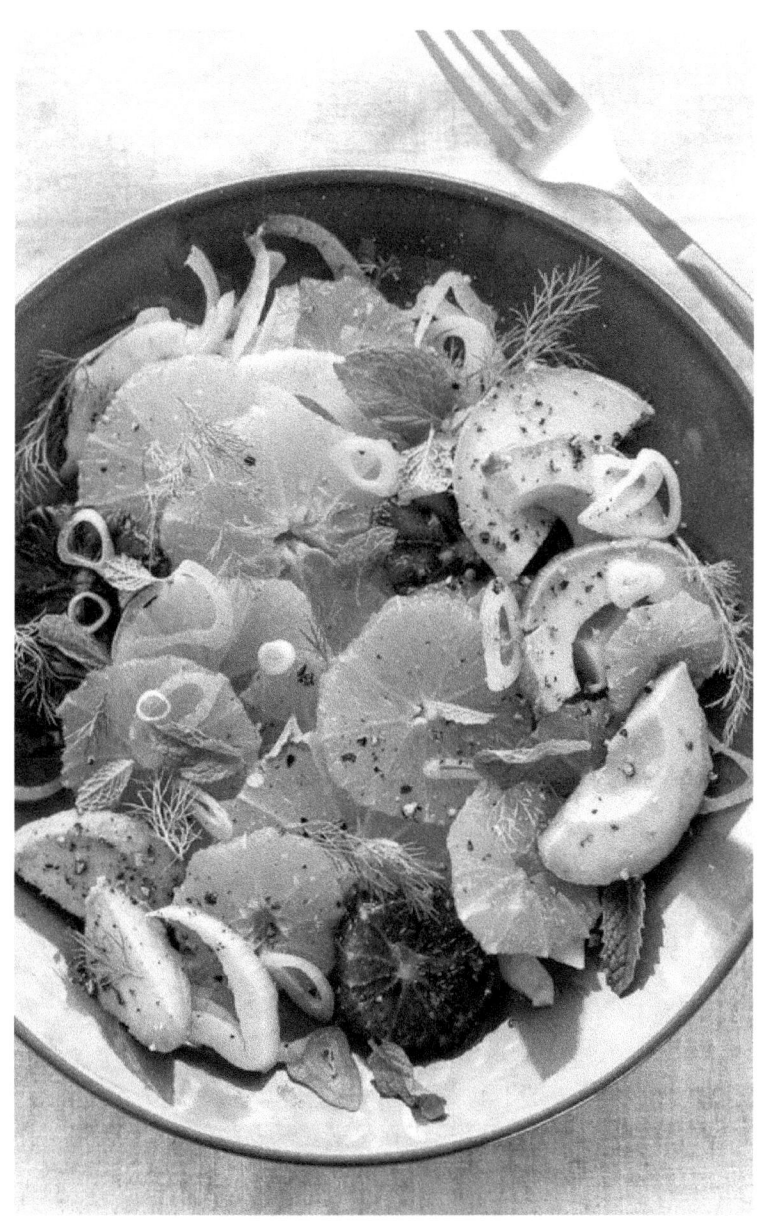

Chapter 2

Main courses

Nuggets of seitan with peppers

PREPARATION TIME: 20 minutes
COOKING TIME: 20 minutes
CALORIES: 305

INGREDIENTS FOR 4 SERVINGS
- 400 grams of seitan
- 2 shallots
- 1 red pepper
- 1 yellow pepper
- 2 bay leaves
- Oatmeal to taste
- Salt and pepper to taste
- 100 ml of vegetable broth
- Olive oil to taste

DIRECTIONS
1. Remove the cap from the peppers, then remove the seeds and white filaments and wash them. Finally cut them into strips.
2. Rinse and pat the seitan with absorbent paper and then cut it into cubes.
3. Peel and wash the shallots and then cut them into slices.

4. Wash and dry the bay leaves.
5. Put the oatmeal on a plate and pass the seitan cubes over the flour.
6. Heat two tablespoons of oil in a pan and as soon as it is hot, put the seitan to brown for 4 minutes.
7. Now add the peppers, shallots and bay leaf.
8. Season with salt and pepper, add the broth and then cover the pan with a lid.
9. Cook for another 15 minutes.
10. As soon as it is cooked, put the seitan and the vegetables on the plates, sprinkle it with the cooking juices and serve.

Sandwich with flavoured tofu

PREPARATION TIME: 20 minutes
COOKING TIME: 3 minutes

CALORIES: 211

INGREDIENTS FOR 4 SERVINGS
- 8 slices of wholemeal bread
- 150 grams of tofu
- 4 lettuce leaves
- 2 tomatoes
- 1 yellow pepper
- 1 sprig of chopped parsley
- Salt and pepper to taste
- Olive oil to taste

DIRECTIONS
1. Wash the pepper, cut them in half and remove seeds and white filaments. Now cut it into strips.
2. Wash the tomatoes and then cut them into slices.
3. Wash and dry the lettuce and then cut it into small pieces.
4. Rinse and pat the tofu with absorbent paper. Now cut it into cubes.
5. Heat a tablespoon of oil in a pan and when hot, sauté the tofu for 3 minutes.
6. Put the tofu in a bowl and mash it with a fork.
7. Add the chopped basil, salt and pepper and mix well.

8. Now put the bread to toast in the toaster.
9. As soon as the bread is ready, spread half of it with the flavoured tofu.
10. Put the pepper on top, then the tomato and finally the lettuce.
11. Close with the other half of the bread, place on plates and serve.

Amaranth and pumpkin croquettes

PREPARATION TIME: 20 minutes

COOKING TIME: 40 minutes
CALORIES: 330

INGREDIENTS FOR 4 SERVINGS
- 150 grams of amaranth
- 2 medium sized potatoes
- 2 shallots
- 250 grams of pumpkin
- 1 clove of garlic
- 1 sprig of chopped parsley
- Oatmeal to taste
- Olive oil to taste
- Salt and pepper to taste

DIRECTIONS
1. Peel the potatoes and then wash them thoroughly. Cut the potatoes into cubes.
2. Wash the pumpkin pulp and then grate it.
3. Peel the shallots, wash and chop them.
4. Peel and wash the garlic and then chop it.
5. In a pan, heat two tablespoons of oil and as soon as it is hot enough add the shallot.
6. Brown it for a couple of minutes and then add the potatoes and pumpkin.

7. Season with salt, pepper, and cook for 15 minutes.
8. Now add the amaranth and 450 ml of water and cook for another 20 minutes.
9. Now add the minced garlic, parsley, and mix.
10. Turn off and let cool.
11. When the mixture is cold enough, take small quantities and make meatballs.
12. Put the oatmeal on a plate and pass the meatballs over it.
13. Heat a tablespoon of oil in a pan and when hot, cook the meatballs for 3 minutes per side.
14. As soon as they are ready, put them on plates and serve.

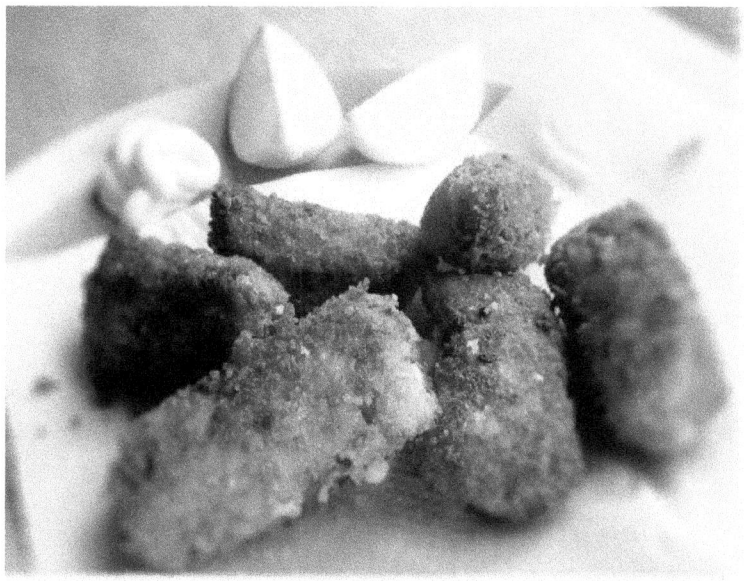

Salad with tofu, pear and honey

PREPARATION TIME: 10 minutes

CALORIES: 180

INGREDIENTS FOR 4 SERVINGS
- 2 small pears
- A stick of celery
- 50 grams of rocket
- 100 grams of grilled tofu
- 8 green peppercorns
- 1 tablespoon of honey
- Olive oil to taste
- Salt and pepper to taste

DIRECTIONS
1. Take the tofu and cut it into cubes. Put it in a bowl with the honey and green pepper. Stir to flavour well.
2. Wash and dry the rocket and place it in the bottom of 4 serving dishes.
3. Wash the celery and then cut it into cubes. Divide it in the plates.
4. Peel the pears, wash them, remove the seeds and then cut them into cubes. Also, divide the pears on the plates.
5. Season the dishes with oil, salt and pepper.
6. Place the tofu cubes in the centre of each plate and serve.

Cucumber, watermelon and mozzarella plant based salad

PREPARATION TIME: 10 minutes
CALORIES: 111

INGREDIENTS FOR 4 SERVINGS

- 1 small watermelon
- 1 cucumber
- 1 vegan mozzarella
- Salt and pepper to taste
- Olive oil to taste
- Tufts of dill to taste

DIRECTIONS

1. Peel the watermelon, remove all the seeds and then cut it into cubes.
2. Wash the cucumber and cut it into slices.
3. Put the cucumber and watermelon in a salad bowl.
4. Cut the mozzarella into cubes and put it in the salad bowl.
5. Season everything with oil, salt, pepper, and the sprigs of dill.
6. Stir to flavour everything well and serve.

Apple and fennel salad

PREPARATION TIME: 15 minutes

CALORIES: 87

INGREDIENTS FOR 4 SERVINGS
- 1 fennel
- 1 apple
- 8 walnuts
- Half a lemon
- Olive oil to taste
- Salt and pepper to taste

DIRECTIONS
1. Remove the beard and the harder outer leaves from the fennel.
2. Wash it and then cut it into slices.
3. Peel the apple, wash it, remove the seeds and cut it into slices.
4. Chop the walnuts with a knife.
5. Put the fennel, walnuts and apples in a salad bowl and mix gently.
6. In a bowl, emulsify together the lemon juice, 2 tablespoons of olive oil, salt and pepper.
7. Sprinkle the salad with the emulsion, mix to flavour well and serve.

Mixed vegetable and fruit salad with chia seeds

PREPARATION TIME: 15 minutes
CALORIES: 66

INGREDIENTS FOR 4 SERVINGS
- 4 lettuce leaves
- 12 cherry tomatoes
- 1 green apple
- A teaspoon of Chia seeds
- Balsamic vinegar to taste
- Salt and pepper to taste
- Olive oil to taste

DIRECTIONS
1. Wash and dry the lettuce leaves.
2. Wash the cherry tomatoes and cut them in half.
3. Wash the apple with all the peel, cut it in half, remove the seeds and then cut it into slices.
4. Put the cherry tomatoes, lettuce and apple in a salad bowl.
5. In a bowl, emulsify together the oil, balsamic vinegar, salt and pepper.
6. Sprinkle the salad with the emulsion and mix to flavour well.
7. Sprinkle the salad with Chia seeds and serve.

Greek salad with tofu

PREPARATION TIME: 15 minutes
CALORIES: 250

INGREDIENTS FOR 4 SERVINGS

- 2 cucumbers
- 20 black olives
- 1 green pepper
- 1 red onion
- 4 tomatoes
- 3 tablespoons of apple cider vinegar
- 200 grams of grilled tofu
- 1 teaspoon of dried oregano
- Salt and pepper to taste
- Olive oil to taste

DIRECTIONS

1. Wash the tomatoes, cut them into wedges and then put them in a salad bowl.
2. Remove the top cap from the pepper. Remove seeds and white filaments. Wash it and then cut it into cubes.
3. Peel and wash the onion and then cut it into slices.
4. Wash the cucumbers and then cut them into rings.
5. Put the vegetables inside the salad bowl.
6. Cut the tofu into cubes and put it together with the vegetables.
7. Finally add the olives and season with vinegar, oil, salt and pepper.
8. Gently mix to flavour everything well.
9. Sprinkle the salad with oregano and serve.

Chickpea and mushroom salad

PREPARATION TIME: 15 minutes
CALORIES: 122

INGREDIENTS FOR 4 SERVINGS
- 400 grams of cooked chickpeas
- 8 lettuce leaves
- 60 grams of mushrooms
- 8 cherry tomatoes
- 2 lemons
- Olive oil to taste
- Salt and pepper to taste

DIRECTIONS
1. Wash the cherry tomatoes and then cut them in half.
2. Wash and dry the lettuce and then cut them into slices.
3. Remove the earthy part of the mushrooms, rinse them under running water and then dry them. Cut them into thin slices.
4. Put the mushrooms, cherry tomatoes and lettuce in a salad bowl.
5. Now add the chickpeas and mix.
6. Wash and dry the lemons and then cut one into rings. Strain the juice of the other into a bowl.
7. Put the lemon slices in the salad bowl with the other vegetables.
8. In the bowl with the lemon juice, add oil, salt and pepper. Mix well to obtain a homogeneous emulsion.
9. Pour the emulsion over the salad, mix well and then serve.

Onion and walnut plum cake

PREPARATION TIME: 30 minutes+3 hours to rest
COOKING TIME: 30 minutes

CALORIES: 680

INGREDIENTS FOR 4 SERVINGS
- 400 grams of oat flour
- 100 grams of spelt flour
- 25 grams of brewer's yeast
- 120 grams of shelled walnuts
- 1 white onion
- 1 teaspoon of salt

DIRECTIONS
1. Peel and wash the onion and then chop it.
2. Take 60 grams of walnuts and chop them.
3. Break up the yeast with your hands and put it in a bowl with 300 ml of water.
4. Gradually add the flour, salt and start kneading.
5. Knead well until you get a smooth and lump-free dough.
6. Form the dough into a ball and let it rise covered with cling film for an hour.
7. After the hour, reshuffle the dough for a short time and let it rise for another hour.
8. Now put the dough on a lightly floured work surface and roll it out in the shape of a rectangle.

9. Put the onions and walnuts in the centre of the dough.
10. Roll the dough on itself.
11. Take a plum cake mold and line it with parchment paper.
12. Put the dough inside and cover it with cling film. Let it rise for another hour.
13. After the hour, remove the film and sprinkle the surface with the rest of the walnuts.
14. Put the mold in the oven and cook at 220 ° C for 35 minutes.
15. After the cooking time, remove from the oven and let the plum cake cool.
16. Now remove from the mold, cut and into slices and serve.

Eggplant, tomatoes and plant based mozzarella

PREPARATION TIME: 20 minutes

COOKING TIME: 10 minutes
CALORIES: 237

INGREDIENTS FOR 4 SERVINGS
- 2 eggplants
- 4 tomatoes
- 2 plant based mozzarella
- 2 cloves of garlic
- 1 teaspoon of oregano
- Olive oil to taste
- Salt and pepper to taste

DIRECTIONS
1. Wash the aubergines and then cut them into thin slices.
2. Heat a grill. When it is hot, put the eggplants and grill.
3. Meanwhile, wash the tomatoes and then cut them into slices.
4. Peel and wash the garlic cloves and then chop them.
5. Cut the mozzarella into slices.
6. In a bowl, mix together the minced garlic and oregano.
7. Now put the aubergines on a serving dish, then the tomatoes and finally the mozzarella.
8. Season with oil, salt and pepper.
9. Sprinkle everything with the oregano and garlic mix and serve.

Baked seitan with capers, lemon and mint

PREPARATION TIME: 15 minutes+30 minutes to rest
COOKING TIME: 10 minutes

CALORIES: 320

INGREDIENTS FOR 4 SERVINGS
- 600 grams of seitan
- 2 cloves of garlic
- 300 ml of vegetable broth
- 1 shallot
- 1 tablespoon of capers
- 2 lemons
- 12 mint leaves
- Olive oil to taste
- Salt and pepper to taste

DIRECTIONS
1. Rinse the seitan and pat it dry with absorbent paper.
2. Now put the seitan in a bowl.
3. Wash and dry the mint leaves.
4. Peel and wash the garlic cloves and the shallot and then cut them into slices.
5. Put 6 mint leaves, garlic, shallot, salt, pepper and two tablespoons of oil in the bowl with the seitan.
6. Cover the bowl and leave to marinate for 30 minutes.
7. After 30 minutes, drain the seitan and then cut it into slices.

8. Brush a baking sheet with olive oil and then put the slices of seitan at the bottom.
9. Wash and dry the lemons and then cut them into rings.
10. Place the lemon slices on top of the seitan.
11. Sprinkle with the capers and mint leaves and season with oil, salt and pepper.
12. Add the broth and then put in the oven to cook at 190°C for 10 minutes.
13. After the cooking time, take the seitan out of the oven and let it rest for 2 minutes.
14. Put the seitan and lemons on the plates, sprinkle with the cooking juices and serve.

Juniper and orange seitan

PREPARATION TIME: 12 minutes
COOKING TIME: 10 minutes
CALORIES: 165

INGREDIENTS FOR 4 SERVINGS
- 600 grams of seitan
- 6 juniper berries
- 1 orange
- Oatmeal to taste
- 30 grams of soy butter
- Salt and pepper to taste

DIRECTIONS
1. Rinse the seitan and pat it dry with absorbent paper, then cut it into slices.
2. Put some oatmeal on a plate and flour the slices of seitan.
3. Wash the orange, remove the zest and strain the juice into a bowl.
4. Put the butter in a pan and as soon as it has melted, add the juniper berries and orange zest.
5. Toast for a couple of minutes, and then add the slices of seitan.
6. Brown them for 2 minutes on each side and then add salt, pepper and orange juice.
7. Continue cooking for another 5 minutes and then turn off.
8. Put the slices on serving plates, sprinkle them with the cooking juices and serve.

Seitan with herbs

PREPARATION TIME: 10 minutes

COOKING TIME: 8 minutes
CALORIES: 250

INGREDIENTS FOR 4 SERVINGS
- 400 grams of seitan
- 4 juniper berries
- 4 sage leaves
- 4 bay leaves
- 1 sprig of rosemary
- 1 sprig of thyme
- 1 tablespoon of chopped chives
- 1 tablespoon of green peppercorns
- Salt and pepper to taste
- Olive oil to taste

DIRECTIONS
1. Wash sage, thyme, rosemary and bay leaves and then chop them.
2. Put the herbs on a plate. Add the green pepper, 2 tablespoons of olive oil, salt, pepper, and mix.
3. Rinse and dab the seitan and then cut it into thin slices.
4. Pass it over the herb mixture on both sides.
5. Heat a grill and as soon as it is hot, put the seitan to grill, 4 minutes per side.
6. Put the slices of seitan on the plates and serve immediately.

Strips of tempeh with olives

PREPARATION TIME: 10 minutes

COOKING TIME: 10 minutes
CALORIES: 190

INGREDIENTS FOR 4 SERVINGS
- 400 grams of tempeh
- 300 grams of cherry tomatoes
- 100 grams of black olives
- 1 teaspoon of dried oregano
- Olive oil to taste
- Salt and pepper to taste

DIRECTIONS
1. Rinse and pat the tempeh with absorbent paper and then cut it into strips.
2. Wash the cherry tomatoes and then cut them into four wedges.
3. Heat two tablespoons of oil in a pan and as soon as it is hot, add the cherry tomatoes.
4. Sauté them for two minutes and then add the tempeh.
5. Cook for 3 minutes. Season with salt and pepper, mix and finally add the olives.
6. Continue cooking for another two minutes. Turn off and sprinkle everything with oregano.
7. Now put the tempeh and the vegetables on the plates and serve.

Fried tofu with lemon

PREPARATION TIME: 10 minutes+30 minutes of rest
COOKING TIME: 10 minutes
CALORIES: 202

INGREDIENTS FOR 4 SERVINGS
- 400 grams of tofu
- 1 shallot
- 1 lemon
- Oatmeal to taste
- Salt and pepper to taste
- Olive oil to taste

DIRECTIONS
1. Rinse the tofu and then pat it dry with absorbent paper.
2. Peel and wash the shallot and then cut it into slices.
3. Wash and dry the lemon and then grate the zest.
4. Put the tofu in a bowl together with the shallot, lemon zest, salt, pepper and two tablespoons of olive oil. Gently mix to flavour better.
5. Leave to marinate for 30 minutes.
6. After 30 minutes, drain the tofu and cut it into cubes.
7. Put the oatmeal on a plate and then pass the tofu cubes in the flour.
8. Put the contents of the bowl with the marinade in a pan and cook for 3 minutes.
9. Now add the tofu cubes and cook until the outside of the tofu is golden brown.

10. Season with salt and pepper, stir one last time and turn off.
11. Put the tofu on serving plates, sprinkle with the cooking juices and serve.

Ginger glazed tofu

PREPARATION TIME: 15 minutes

COOKING TIME: 10 minutes
CALORIES: 248

INGREDIENTS FOR 4 SERVINGS
- 480 grams of tofu
- 1 chilli
- 1 shallot
- 1 star anise
- 2 tablespoons of soy sauce
- 20 grams of fresh grated ginger
- 1 tablespoon of vegan brown sugar
- 10 grams of corn starch
- Olive oil to taste
- Salt and pepper to taste

DIRECTIONS
1. Rinse the tofu and then pat it dry with absorbent paper.
2. Brush a baking sheet with olive oil and put the tofu inside.
3. Peel and wash the shallot and then cut it into slices.
4. Put the star anise and the shallot inside the pan.
5. Sprinkle with ginger, salt and pepper and sprinkle everything with olive oil.
6. Put the baking sheet in the oven and cook at 200 ° C for 10 minutes.

7. After 10 minutes, remove from the oven and transfer the tofu to a serving dish.
8. Put the cooking juices in a saucepan.
9. Wash and chop the chilli and put it in the saucepan with the cooking juices.
10. Also, add the sugar, soy sauce, corn starch and a ladle of warm water.
11. Cook over medium heat until the sauce thickens.
12. Sprinkle the tofu with the sauce, cut into slices and serve.

Quiche with potatoes, zucchini and plant based mozzarella

PREPARATION TIME: 20 minutes

COOKING TIME: 25 minutes
CALORIES: 348

INGREDIENTS FOR 4 SERVINGS
- 250 grams of plant based puff pastry
- 280 grams of potatoes
- 1 large zucchini
- 1 clove of garlic
- 120 grams of plant based mozzarella
- Salt and pepper to taste
- Olive oil to taste

DIRECTIONS
1. Start with the potatoes. Peel them, wash them thoroughly and then cut them into cubes.
2. Heat a tablespoon of olive oil and then put the potatoes to brown for 5 minutes. Season with salt and pepper and turn off.
3. Peel and wash the garlic and then chop it.
4. Wash the zucchini and then cut them into cubes.
5. Put a tablespoon of olive oil in another pan and when it is hot, put the garlic to brown.
6. Add the zucchini, mix, season with salt, pepper, and cook for 5 minutes.
7. Cut the mozzarella into cubes.

8. Brush a round baking pan with olive oil.
9. Cover it with the puff pastry.
10. Put the potatoes, zucchini and mozzarella inside.
11. Put in the oven and cook at 200 ° C for 20 minutes.
12. When it is cooked, remove the quiche from the oven and let it rest for a couple of minutes.
13. Cut it into slices, put it on serving plates and serve.

Quiche with cherry tomatoes, vegan mozzarella and capers

PREPARATION TIME: 10 minutes
COOKING TIME: 20 minutes

CALORIES: 383

INGREDIENTS FOR 4 SERVINGS
- 300 grams of plant based puffy pastry
- 200 grams of vegan mozzarella
- 12 cherry tomatoes
- 1 tablespoon of capers
- 1 tablespoon of chopped chives
- Olive oil to taste
- Salt and pepper to taste

DIRECTIONS
1. Brush a round baking pan and line it with the puff pastry.
2. Wash and dry the cherry tomatoes and then cut them in half.
3. Cut the mozzarella into cubes.
4. Put the cherry tomatoes and mozzarella inside the puff pastry.
5. Season with oil, salt, pepper, and then sprinkle with capers and chives.
6. Put the baking sheet in the oven and cook at 200 ° C for 20 minutes.
7. After 20 minutes, remove from the oven, let it rest for a couple of minutes then cut it into slices and serve.

Quiche with vegetables

PREPARATION TIME: 20 minutes

COOKING TIME: 50 minutes
CALORIES: 375

INGREDIENTS FOR 4 SERVINGS
- 250 grams of puff pastry
- 300 ml of plant based béchamel
- 2 carrots
- 1 onion
- 100 grams of spinach
- 50 grams of peas
- Olive oil to taste
- Salt and pepper to taste

DIRECTIONS
1. Peel and wash the carrots and then cut them into slices.
2. Peel and wash the onion and then cut it into slices.
3. Wash and drain the peas and spinach.
4. Bring a pot of water and salt to a boil and then cook the onion, carrots and peas for 15 minutes.
5. After 15 minutes, add the spinach and continue for another 5 minutes.
6. Turn off, drain the vegetables and let them cool.
7. Brush a baking sheet with olive oil and then line it with the puff pastry.
8. Put the vegetables in a bowl and add the béchamel and pepper.

9. Mix everything well and then put it inside the puff pastry.
10. Put in the oven and cook at 200 ° C for 35 minutes.
11. As soon as it is cooked, take it out of the oven and let it cool down.
12. Cut the quiche into slices, place on serving plates and serve.

Quiche with zucchini, zucchini flowers and plant based mozzarella

PREPARATION TIME: 20 minutes
COOKING TIME: 35 minutes
CALORIES: 409

INGREDIENTS FOR 4 SERVINGS
- 250 grams of plant-based puff pastry
- 500 grams of zucchini
- 2 plant based mozzarella
- 50 ml of soymilk cream
- 6 zucchini flowers
- 1 clove of garlic
- Olive oil to taste
- Salt and pepper to taste

DIRECTIONS
1. Wash the zucchinis and then cut them into slices.
2. Wash the zucchini flowers, dry them and then cut them into strips.
3. Peel and wash the garlic clove and then chop it.
4. Put a tablespoon of olive oil in a pan and when it is hot, put the garlic to brown.
5. Put the zucchinis, mix, and season with salt, pepper, and cook for 10 minutes.
6. Put the cream, salt and pepper in a bowl and mix.
7. Add the zucchinis and mix.

8. Brush a baking sheet with olive oil and then line it with the puff pastry.
9. Pour the mixture with the zucchini inside.
10. Place the zucchini flowers and the sliced mozzarella on top.
11. Put the pan in the oven and cook at 180 ° C for 20 minutes.
12. After the cooking time, take the quiche out of the oven, let it cool, then cut into slices and serve.

Potato, pumpkin and plant based mozzarella pie

PREPARATION TIME: 20 minutes

COOKING TIME: 50 minutes
CALORIES: 234

INGREDIENTS FOR 4 SERVINGS
- 300 grams of potatoes
- 3 vegan mozzarella
- 200 grams of pumpkin pulp
- Olive oil to taste
- Salt and pepper to taste

DIRECTIONS
1. Peel the potatoes, wash them thoroughly and then cut them into thin slices.
2. Peel and remove the seeds from the pumpkin. Wash it and then cut it into slices.
3. Cut the mozzarella into thin slices.
4. Take a baking dish and brush the bottom with olive oil.
5. First, put the potatoes, season with oil, salt and pepper and then add the mozzarella.
6. Now put the pumpkin, season with oil, salt and pepper and finish with the remaining mozzarella.
7. Put the dish in the oven and cook at 180 ° C for 50 minutes.
8. When the pie is cooked, take it out of the oven and let it cool for 5 minutes.
9. Cut the pie into 4 parts, put it on serving plates and serve.

Baked pumpkin, chickpeas and tofu

PREPARATION TIME: 15 minutes
COOKING TIME: 35 minutes
CALORIES: 179

INGREDIENTS FOR 4 SERVINGS
- 500 grams of pumpkin
- 250 grams of cooked chickpeas
- 120 grams of tofu
- 2 sprigs of rosemary
- Olive oil to taste
- Salt and pepper to taste

DIRECTIONS
1. Peel the pumpkin, remove the seeds, wash it and then cut it into slices.
2. Take a baking sheet and line it with parchment paper.
3. Put the pumpkin slices inside the baking tray.
4. Add the chickpeas.
5. Wash and dry the rosemary and take only the needles.
6. Sprinkle the pumpkin and chickpeas with the rosemary needles.
7. Season with oil, salt, pepper, and cook in the oven at 190 ° for 30 minutes.
8. Meanwhile, rinse the tofu and pat it dry with absorbent paper, then cut it into cubes.
9. Remove the squash from the oven and add the tofu cubes.
10. Return to the oven and continue cooking for another 5 minutes.

11. Now take out of the oven, put the pumpkin with the tofu and chickpeas on the serving plates and serve.

Roast seitan with apples

PREPARATION TIME: 15 minutes

COOKING TIME: 15 minutes
CALORIES: 324

INGREDIENTS FOR 4 SERVINGS
- 400 grams of seitan
- 4 yellow apples
- 1 orange
- 30 grams of soy butter
- 1 teaspoon of cinnamon
- 1 teaspoon of honey
- Olive oil to taste
- Salt and pepper to taste

DIRECTIONS
1. Peel the apples, wash them and cut them in half. Remove the seeds and then cut them into thin slices.
2. Wash and dry the orange, grate the zest and strain the juice into a bowl.
3. Rinse the seitan and then pat it dry with absorbent paper.
4. Take a baking sheet and put the seitan inside.
5. Season it with oil, salt and pepper and put it to cook in the oven at 180 ° C for 10 minutes.
6. Meanwhile, put the butter in a pan to melt.
7. As soon as it is melted, add the apples with the orange juice and the grated zest.

8. Add a glass of water, honey and cinnamon and cook until they are very soft.
9. As soon as they are ready, turn them off and blend them with an immersion blender until you get a smooth and homogeneous cream.
10. When the seitan is cooked, take it out of the oven and let it rest for 5 minutes. Then cut it into slices.
11. Put the apple custard in the bottom of the serving plates and over the slices of seitan and serve.

Green beans, potatoes and tofu

PREPARATION TIME: 20 minutes
COOKING TIME: 35 minutes

CALORIES: 153

INGREDIENTS FOR 4 SERVINGS
- 250 grams of green beans
- 100 grams of tofu
- 300 grams of potatoes
- 300 grams of cherry tomatoes
- Half onion
- 1 clove of garlic
- Olive oil to taste
- Salt and pepper to taste

DIRECTIONS
1. Peel and wash the potatoes thoroughly and then cut them into cubes.
2. Peel the garlic and onion and then chop them.
3. Wash the cherry tomatoes and cut them in half.
4. Check the green beans and then wash them.
5. Put a tablespoon of oil to heat in a pan and then add onion and garlic to brown.
6. Now add the potatoes and cook for 6 minutes.
7. Now add the cherry tomatoes and cook for another 5 minutes.
8. Finally add the green beans and continue cooking for another 25

minutes.
9. Stir occasionally and a couple of minutes before the end of cooking season with salt and pepper.
10. While the vegetables are cooking, pat the tofu with paper towels.
11. Heat a grill and when hot, grill the tofu for 5 minutes on each side.
12. Remove it from the grill and cut it into cubes.
13. As soon as they are cooked, turn off the vegetables and put them on the plates.
14. Place the tofu cubes on top and serve.

Vegetable cream buns

PREPARATION TIME: 20 minutes
COOKING TIME: 10 minutes

CALORIES: 405

INGREDIENTS FOR 4 SERVINGS
- 4 wholemeal hamburger buns
- 1 carrot
- 1 onion
- 1 red pepper
- 150 grams of plant based ricotta
- 60 grams of plant based mayonnaise
- Olive oil to taste
- Salt and parsley to taste

DIRECTIONS
1. Peel and wash the carrot and onion and then cut them into slices.
2. Cut the pepper in half. Remove seeds and white filaments. Wash it and cut it into slices.
3. Heat a tablespoon of oil in a pan and as soon as it is hot, brown the vegetables.
4. Stir, season with salt, pepper, and cook for 10 minutes.
5. After 10 minutes, turn off and let the vegetables cool.
6. As soon as they are cold, put them in a bowl.
7. Add the ricotta and mayonnaise and mix to flavour everything well.
8. Cut the buns in half, stuff them with the vegetable cream, close them and serve.

Tofu and almond meatballs

PREPARATION TIME: 20 minutes
COOKING TIME: 5 minutes

CALORIES: 263

INGREDIENTS FOR 4 SERVINGS
- 500 grams of tofu
- 40 grams of already skinned almonds
-
- Soy sauce to taste
- White sesame seeds to taste
- Olive oil to taste
- Salt and pepper to taste

DIRECTIONS
1. Rinse and pat the tofu with absorbent paper.
2. Cut it into cubes and sauté it in a pan with olive oil for 5 minutes.
3. Season with salt and pepper, stir and then turn off.
4. Now put the tofu in a bowl.
5. Mash the tofu with a fork. Now add the soy sauce and mix well.
6. Chop the almonds and then put them in the bowl with the tofu.
7. Mix well and then form meatballs by taking a little of the mixture at a time.
8. Put the sesame in a non-stick pan and toast it.
9. Now put the sesame on a plate and pass over the tofu balls.
10. The tofu meatballs are ready, put them on the plates and serve.

Follow a plant-based meal plan regularly to live better in strength and health every day of your life.

Carolyn J. Perez

Plant-Based Diet

Lose weight and get back in shape by following easy and delicious Plant-Based recipes

Carolyn J. Perez

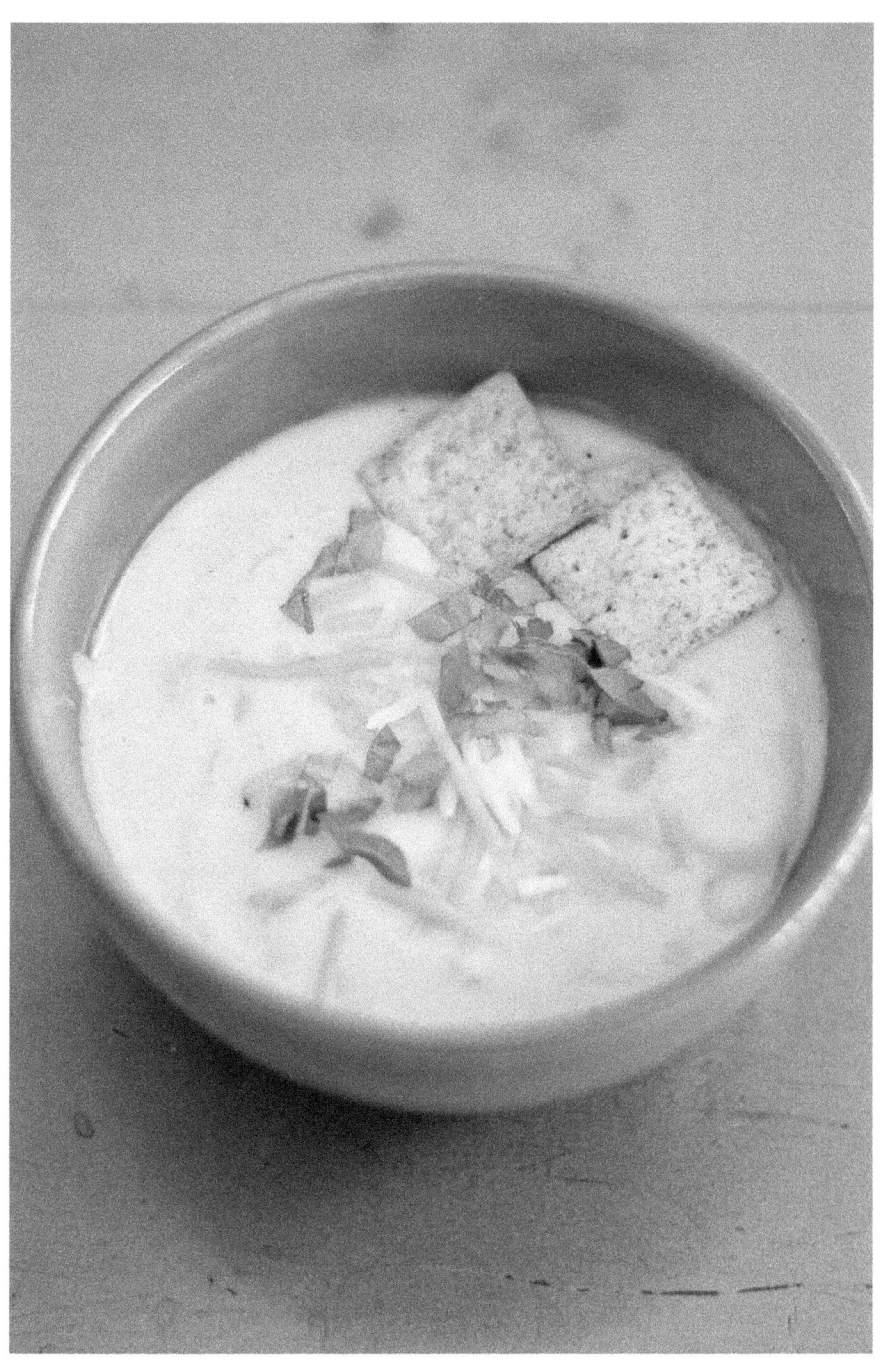

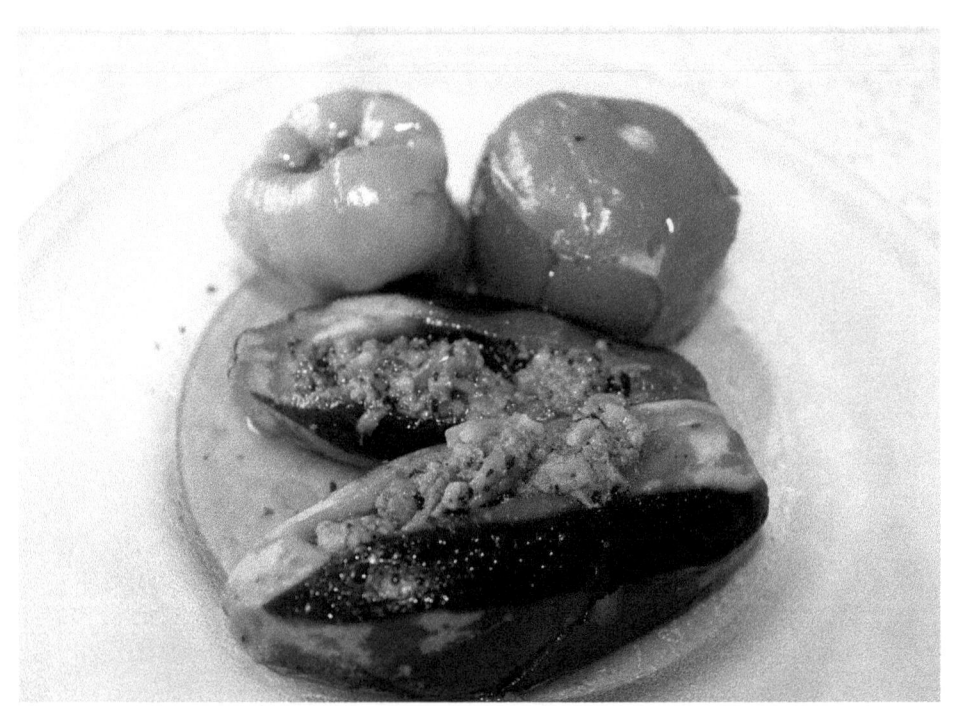

© **Copyright 2021 - All rights reserved.**

The content contained within this book may not be reproduced, duplicated or transmitted without direct written permission from the author or the publisher.

Under no circumstances will any blame or legal responsibility be held against the publisher, or author, for any damages, reparation, or monetary loss due to the information contained within this book. Either directly or indirectly.

Legal Notice:

This book is copyright protected. This book is only for personal use. You cannot amend, distribute, sell, use, quote or paraphrase any part, or the content within this book, without the consent of the author or publisher.

Disclaimer Notice:

Please note the information contained within this document is for educational and entertainment purposes only. All effort has been executed to present accurate, up to date, and reliable, complete information. No warranties of any kind are declared or implied. Readers acknowledge that the author is not engaging in the rendering of legal, financial, medical or professional advice. The content within this book has been derived from various sources. Please consult a licensed professional before attempting any techniques outlined in this book.

By reading this document, the reader agrees that under no circumstances is the author responsible for any losses, direct or indirect, which are incurred as a result of the use of information contained within this document, including, but not limited to, — errors, omissions, or inaccuracies.

Contents

INTRODUCTION.. 118

PLANT BASED DIET: WHAT ARE WE TALKING ABOUT?................... 120

MAIN DIFFERENCES BETWEEN VEGAN AND PLANT BASED DIET 122

    Spelt spaghetti with carrots, tofu and parsley 130
    Rice noodles with coriander pesto 132
    Whole wheat spaghetti with tomato, garlic and chilli.............. 134
    Whole wheat pasta with rocket sauce 136
    Potatoes gnocchi with cabbage and hazelnuts 138
    Potatoes gnocchi with zucchini and tomatoes 140
    Eggplant and mint Couscous 142
    Olives melon and tofu Couscous 143
    Veggies Couscous.. 145

  RICE RECIPES 147
    Brown rice with pumpkin and sage.. 147
    Brown rice with walnuts... 149
    Cherry tomato curry and black rice 151
    Brown rice with cherry tomatoes and vegan............................ 153
    mozzarella... 153
    Brown rice with spinach and raisins.. 155
    Brown rice with spinach and raisins.. 157
    Black rice with tofu, broad beans and cherry 159
    tomatoes... 159
    Vegetarian Buddha bowl.. 162
    Beetroot brown rice 164
    Brown rice with watermelon and tofu 166
    Black rice with pumpkin and pears 168
    Wholemeal risotto with saffron 170
    Brown rice with leeks, apples and curry................................... 172
    Brown rice with tomato and herbs 174
    Black rice salad with mixed vegetables and pine 176
    nuts... 176
    Brown rice with lentils 178
    Black rice with peas cream 180

  SOUP RECIPES 182
    Board beans cream 182
    Peas cream.. 184
    Lentils stewed with peppers and shallots................................. 186

Sweet potato soup	188
Bean and cabbage soup	190
Soup with red onion	192
Basil soup	194
Cream of onions	196
Cold cream of peppers and tofu	198
Potato and carrot soup	200
Chickpea, leek and rosemary soup	202
Spelt soup and porcini mushrooms	204
Zucchini and spinach soup	206
Lentil, oat and nut soup	208
Corn chowder	210
Lentil soup with cumin and lemon	212
Carrot cream and black rice	214
Quinoa and spinach soup	216
Lentil and broccoli soup	218
Cream of tomato soup	220
Carrot, pumpkin and black rice soup	222

Introduction

It is a common thought to think that following a diet is necessarily linked to the concept of actual weight loss. However, this is not always the case: following a diet is often directly linked to the foods that we decide to include in our tables daily.

In addition, we do not always choose the best quality ingredients to cook our dishes.

Sometimes we are so rushed and unruly that we forget that we love our bodies. And what better cure than a healthy diet? Following a healthy diet should become more than an imposition or a punishment, but a real lifestyle.

Moreover, this is the Plant-based diet goal: not to impose a restrictive and sometimes impossible diet to follow, but to recreate a diet based on foods of natural origin and above all healthy. Therefore, the plant based represents a real food trend. However, as we will see it is much more than just a fashion trend, but a real lifestyle.

In addition, it is the aim of this text, or rather of this cookbook, to introduce you to the plant based discipline. And we will do it with a few theoretical explanations, just to make you understand what we are talking about and above all how to prepare it: there will be a purely practical part where you will find 800 recipes on the plant based. These recipes will be divided into appetizers, snacks, first and second courses, side dishes and finally a string of plant based desserts.

In the end, you will be spoiled for choice to start following this healthy dietary discipline.

Plant based diet: what are we talking about?

We already mentioned that more than a real weight loss diet the Plant based diet is a food discipline. Food discipline is enjoying great success not only because it is very fashionable, but because it applies such principles that can be perfectly integrated into our daily lives. The plant-based diet is a true approach to life, starting with nutrition: respect for one's health and body, first of all, which is reflected in respect for all forms of life and the planet in general.

As the word itself says, it deals with a food plan based, precisely on what comes from plants. However, simply calling it that way would be too simplistic.

It is a predominantly plant-based diet, but not only. It is not just about consuming vegetables but about taking natural foods: not industrially processed, not treated, and not deriving from the exploitation of resources and animals, preferably zero km.

So it could be a discipline that aims not only at environmental saving but also at the economic one: think about what advantages, in fact, at the level of your pockets you can have if you apply the principle of 0Km and therefore to be able to harvest your vegetables directly from your garden.

Environmental savings do not only mean pollution reduction: the ethical component (present exclusively in the vegan diet, for example) is combined with a strong will to health. This means that the plant based, in addition to not preferring foods that exploit animals, is also based on foods that are especially unprocessed, fresh, healthy, balanced, light, and rich in essential nutrients. In practice, it is a plant-based diet but not vegan / vegetarian, emphasizing the quality and wholesomeness of foods rather than on their moral value, albeit with great attention to sustainability. Such a lifestyle could therefore be of help, not only to our health, but also to create a more sustainable world for future generations.

Main differences between Vegan and Plant based diet

The plant-based diet is often associated with the vegan diet. This is because both plan to include cruelty free foods that do not involve any animal exploitation.

Furthermore, they are associated precisely because they are both predominantly plant-based.

However, there are some pretty obvious differences between these two diets.

First of all, precisely for the reasoning behind the prevalence of plants.

It is well known that even the vegan diet provides a diet based on foods of plant origin: unlike the plant-based diet, however, nothing of animal derivation is allowed, neither direct nor indirect, nor other products - clothing or accessories - which include the exploitation of animals.

No eggs, no milk, no honey, no leather, so to speak, and not only: in its most rigorous meanings, veganism does not even include the use of yeasts, as the bacteria that compose them are indisputably living beings.

A vegan diet can be balanced if the person who leads it knows well the foods and their combinations, the necessary supplements, and their body's reaction to the lack of certain foods.

On the contrary, the Plant-Based diet is on the one hand more relaxed, on the other more stringent.

What does it mean?

This means that it is on the one hand more relaxed because it is plant-based, but not exclusively vegetable: products of animal origin are allowed, in moderate quantities, but under only one condition, namely the excellent quality of the food itself and its certified origin. For example, eggs can be consumed occasionally but only if very fresh, possibly at zero km, from free-range farms where the hens are not exploited but can live outdoors without constraints.

It is also a somewhat more stringent philosophy than veganism precisely for this reason: as long as it is 100% vegetable, the vegan also consumes heavily processed foods, such as industrial fries. Therefore, the vegan can also eat junk foods or snacks. Conversely, plant-based dieters would never admit highly refined foods of this type.

Both dietary approaches are conscious and do not involve the consumption of meat. However, if vegans are driven by ethical reasons, those who follow a plant-based diet also reject everything processed on an industrial level and unhealthy.

A plant-based diet is a diet that aims to eliminate industrially processed foods and, therefore, potentially more harmful to health. It is based on the consumption of fruit and vegetables, whole grains and avoiding (or minimizing) animal products and processed foods. This means that vegan desserts made with refined sugar or bleached flour are also covered.

There is also a substantial difference between the philosophies behind the two diets. As we said in the previous paragraph and above, the ethical component, which is based on the refusal of any food of animal origin, plays a lot in veganism. While for the plant based is not a purely moral and moralistic discourse but on the real thought of being able to keep healthy with the food discipline and be respectful of the environment surrounding us.

Plant based diet full shopping list. What to eat and what to avoid

Now we can examine the complete shopping list of the plant based diet.
Let's briefly summarize the principles on which this particular type of diet is based:

- Emphasizes whole, minimally processed foods.
- Limits or avoids animal products.
- Focuses on plants, including vegetables, fruits, whole grains, legumes, seeds and nuts, which should make up most of what you eat.
- Excludes refined foods, like added sugars, white flour and processed oils.
- Pays special attention to food quality, promoting locally sourced, organic food whenever possible.

As for what you can usually eat, we can say the general consumption of:

- Wholegrain and flours
- extra virgin olive oil

- Seasonal fruit and vegetables: these foods are the basis of every meal.
- In this diet you can also eat sweets but only and exclusively homemade and with controlled raw materials, simple and not very refined, preferably of vegetable origin - for example by replacing milk with soy or rice drinks, and eggs with other natural thickeners such as flaxseed, or simple ripe banana.
- You can also consume nuts and seeds.

As for absolutely forbidden foods, there are all those ready-made and processed:

- ready-made sauces
- chips
- biscuits
- various kinds of snacks
- sugary cereals,
- Spreads, snacks and many other notoriously unhealthy foods.
- Junk food and fast food are therefore absolutely banned
- Sugar beverages

Regarding the complete shopping list:

- Fruits: Berries, citrus fruits, pears, peaches, pineapple, bananas, etc.
- Vegetables: Kale, spinach, tomatoes, broccoli, cauliflower, carrots, asparagus, peppers, etc.
- Starchy vegetables: Potatoes, sweet potatoes, butternut squash, etc.
- Whole grains: Brown rice, rolled oats, spelt, quinoa, brown rice pasta, barley, etc.
- Healthy fats with omega 3: Avocados, olive oil, coconut oil, unsweetened coconut, etc.
- Legumes: Peas, chickpeas, lentils, peanuts, beans, black beans, etc.
- Seeds, nuts and nut butter: Almonds, cashews, macadamia nuts, pumpkin seeds, sunflower seeds, natural peanut butter, tahini, etc.
- Unsweetened plant-based milk: Coconut milk, almond milk, cashew milk, etc.
- Spices, herbs and seasonings: Basil, rosemary, turmeric, curry, black pepper, salt, etc.
- Condiments: Salsa, mustard, nutritional yeast, soy sauce, vinegar, lemon juice, etc.

- Plant-based protein: Tofu, tempeh, seitan, and plant based protein sources or powders with no added sugar or artificial ingredients.
- Beverages: Coffee, tea, sparkling water, etc.

There is the chance to add food of animal origin very rarely, for example if you have specific nutritional needs or if it has been strongly recommended by your doctor. Anyway, if supplementing your plant-based diet with animal products choose quality products from grocery stores or, better yet, purchase them from local farms.

- Eggs: Pasture-raised when possible.
- Poultry: Free-range, organic when possible.
- Beef and pork: Pastured or grass-fed when possible.
- Seafood: Wild-caught from sustainable fisheries when possible.
- Dairy: Organic dairy products from pasture-raised animals whenever possible.

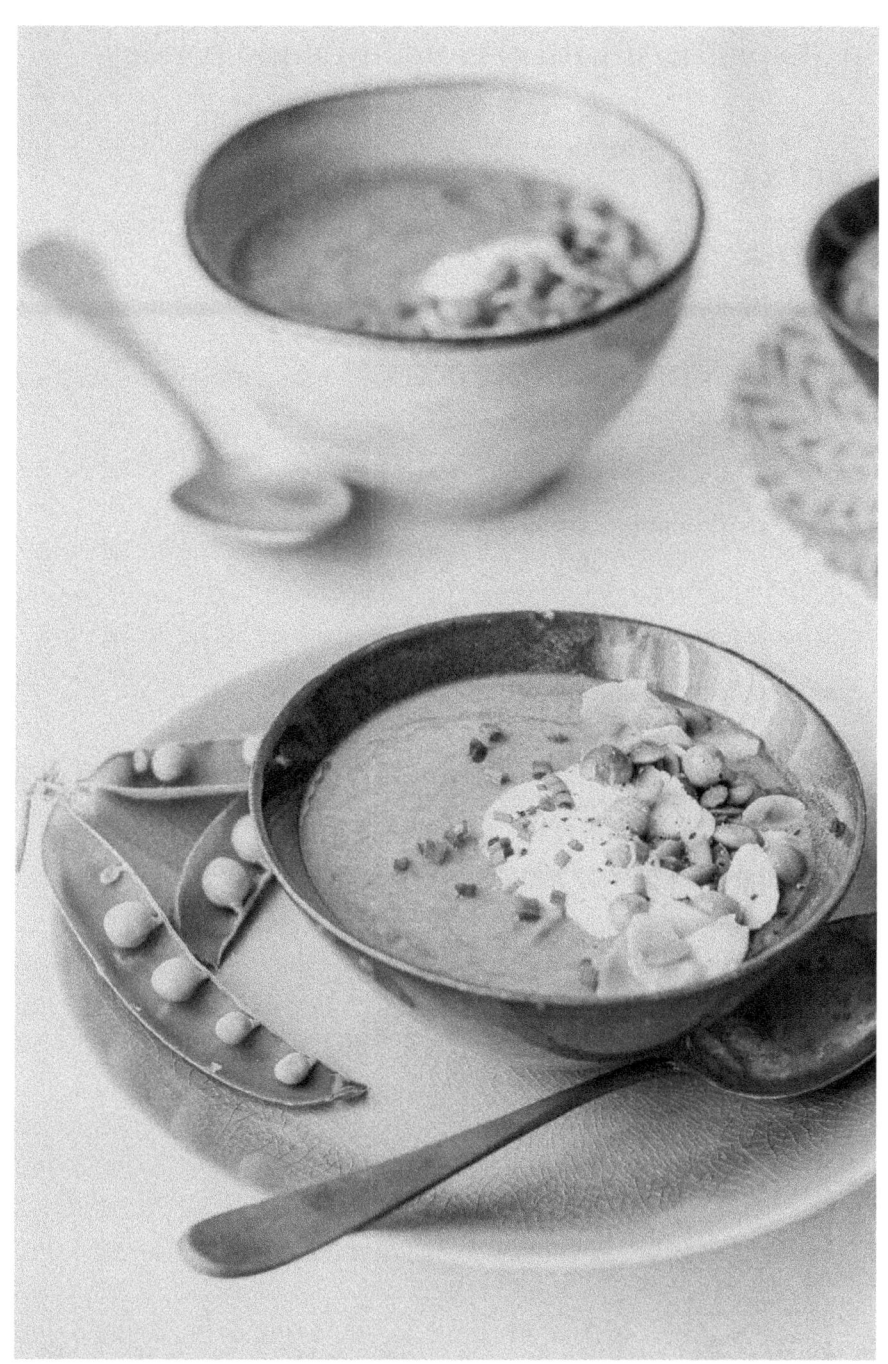

Spelt spaghetti with carrots, tofu and parsley

PREPARATION TIME: 15 minutes

COOKING TIME: 20 minutes
CALORIES: 400

INGREDIENTS FOR 4 SERVINGS
- 320 grams of spelt spaghetti
- 150 grams of grilled tofu
- 2 sprigs of chopped parsley
- olive oil to taste
- Salt and Pepper To Taste.
- a spoonful of sesame seeds

DIRECTIONS
1. Peel and wash the carrots.
2. Cook them in salted boiling water for 8 minutes.
3. Drain them, pass them under running water and then cut them into thin slices.
4. Put a pot with water and salt to boil and as soon as it comes to a boil, put the spaghetti to cook, following the cooking times shown in the package.
5. As soon as it is cooked, drain it and set aside.
6. Heat a little oil in a pan and as soon as it is hot, sauté the carrots for 3 minutes.
7. Add the pasta and sauté for a couple of minutes.
8. Add the sesame seeds, season with salt and pepper, mix well and

turn off.

9. Put the pasta on serving plates, season with the chopped parsley and serve.

Rice noodles with coriander pesto

PREPARATION TIME: 20 minutes
COOKING TIME: 10 minutes
CALORIES: 530

INGREDIENTS FOR 4 SERVINGS
- 320 gr of rice noodles
- 1 lime
- 10 coriander leaves
- 1 green chilli
- 1 red pepper
- 10 basil leaves
- 1 clove of garlic
- 8 shelled walnuts
- Olive oil to taste
- Salt and pepper to taste

DIRECTIONS
1. Wash the coriander and basil leaves.
2. Peel and wash the garlic.
3. Put the garlic, walnuts, coriander and basil in the glass of the blender.
4. Add oil, salt and pepper and blend everything until you get a thick and homogeneous mixture.
5. Put a pot of water and salt to boil and then cook the noodles following the instructions on the package.

6. In the meantime, wash the peppers and then chop them.
7. Drain the noodles and put them in a bowl. Season with the chilli, coriander pesto and lime juice and mix.
8. Put the noodles on the plates and serve.

Whole wheat spaghetti with tomato, garlic and chilli

PREPARATION TIME: 10 minutes

COOKING TIME: 25 minutes
CALORIES: 377

INGREDIENTS FOR 4 SERVINGS
- 320 grams of wholemeal spaghetti
- 2 cloves of garlic
- 2 hot red chillies
- 600 grams of tomato sauce
- Salt to taste
- Olive oil to taste

DIRECTIONS
1. Peel and wash the garlic cloves
2. Wash the peppers, cut them in half, remove the seeds and then cut them into small pieces.
3. Heat some oil in a pan and as soon as it is hot, add the garlic and hot peppers.
4. Sauté them for 2 minutes and then pour the tomato puree.
5. Season with salt, stir, cover with the lid and cook over low heat for 25 minutes.
6. In the meantime, bring salt and water to a boil in a saucepan.
7. Put the pasta to cook following the package directions.
8. When it is ready, drain it and put it in the pan with the tomato.

9. Season, over high heat, for 30 seconds and turn off.
10. Put the spaghetti on serving plates and serve immediately.

Whole wheat pasta with rocket sauce

PREPARATION TIME: minutes
COOKING TIME: minutes

CALORIES: 332

INGREDIENTS FOR 4 SERVINGS
- 320 grams of wholemeal pasta
- 2 onions
- 200 grams of tomato pulp
- 50 grams of rocket
- Olive oil to taste
- Salt and pepper to taste

DIRECTIONS
1. Peel the onions, wash and chop them.
2. Wash and dry the rocket.
3. Heat a drizzle of oil in a pan and as soon as it is hot, put the onion to brown.
4. Now add the tomato pulp, mix, season with salt, pepper, and cook for 15 minutes.
5. In the meantime, prepare the pasta.
6. Boil the water with the salt and when it comes to a boil, cook the pasta.
7. As soon as it is cooked, drain it and keep it temporarily aside.
8. After 15 minutes, add the rocket to the tomato sauce.
9. Mix and cook for a couple of minutes and then add the pasta.

10. Stir, cook for a couple of minutes and then turn off.
11. Put on serving plates and serve.

Potatoes gnocchi with cabbage and hazelnuts

PREPARATION TIME: 10 minutes
COOKING TIME: 20/25 minutes

CALORIES: 586

INGREDIENTS FOR 4 SERVINGS
- 500 grams of homemade potato gnocchi (see basic recipe)
- 1 small cabbage
- 30 grams of chopped hazelnuts
- 1 garlic clove
- Olive oil to taste
- Salt and pepper to taste

DIRECTIONS
1. Wash the cabbage, dry it and then cut it into strips.
2. Peel and wash the garlic and then chop it.
3. Put a tablespoon of oil in a pan and as soon as it is hot, put the garlic to brown.
4. When it is golden brown, sauté the cabbage for 2-3 minutes.
5. Season with salt, pepper, and mix.
6. Cook for another 15 minutes.
7. Meanwhile, put a pot of water and salt to boil.
8. As soon as it comes to a boil, put the gnocchi to cook.
9. The gnocchi will be ready when they rise to the surface.
10. At this point, drain them and put them in the pan with the cabbage.
11. Stir to flavour well and then turn off.

12. Put the gnocchi on the plates, sprinkle them with the chopped hazelnuts and serve.

Potatoes gnocchi with zucchini and tomatoes

PREPARATION TIME: 15 minutes
COOKING TIME: 20 minutes

CALORIES: 538

INGREDIENTS FOR 4 SERVINGS
- 600 grams of homemade potato gnocchi (see basic recipe)
- 1 zucchini
- 200 grams of cherry tomatoes
- 1 clove of garlic
- Olive oil to taste
- Salt and pepper to taste

DIRECTIONS
1. Start by putting a saucepan with plenty of water and salt on the stove and bring it to a boil.
2. Meanwhile, wash the cherry tomatoes and cut them in half.
3. Wash the zucchini and then cut them into cubes.
4. Peel and wash the garlic.
5. Heat a drizzle of oil in a pan and when hot, brown the garlic.
6. As soon as the garlic is golden brown, sauté the tomatoes and zucchini for a couple of minutes. Season with salt and pepper, stir and continue cooking for another 10 minutes.
7. When the water starts to boil, put the gnocchi to cook.
8. The gnocchi will be ready when they all rise to the surface.

9. At this point, drain them and put them in the pan with the zucchini and cherry tomatoes.
10. Stir, cook for a minute and turn off.
11. Put the gnocchi on serving plates and serve.

Eggplant and mint Couscous

PREPARATION TIME: 20 minutes

COOKING TIME: 15 minutes
CALORIES: 154

INGREDIENTS FOR 4 SERVINGS
- 200 grams of couscous
- Half a lemon
- 1 eggplant
- 1 clove of garlic
- 6 mint leaves
- Olive oil to taste
- Salt and pepper to taste

DIRECTIONS
1. Start with the couscous. Bring 400 ml of water to a boil.
2. Put the couscous in a bowl and then cover it with boiling water.
3. Let it sit for 10 minutes.
4. Meanwhile, peel and wash the garlic and then chop it.
5. Wash and dry the mint and then cut it into strips.
6. Wash the eggplant and then cut it into thin slices.
7. Heat a grill and when it is hot, put the eggplant to grill.
8. As soon as it is ready, cut the eggplant slices into strips.
9. After 10 minutes, season the couscous with oil.
10. Mix well and then add the eggplant, garlic and mint.
11. Season with oil, salt and pepper and serve.

Olives melon and tofu Couscous

PREPARATION TIME: 10 minutes
COOKING TIME: 15 minutes

CALORIES: 290

INGREDIENTS FOR 4 SERVINGS
- 300 grams of couscous
- 100 grams of tofu
- 6 black olives
- 6 green olives
- Half a melon
- 4 mint leaves
- A sprig of chopped parsley
- Half a lemon
- Olive oil to taste
- Salt and pepper to taste

DIRECTIONS
1. Start by preparing the couscous. Put the couscous in a bowl.
2. Bring 700 ml of water to a boil and then cover the couscous.
3. Cover the bowl with the couscous and let it rest for 10 minutes.
4. Meanwhile, prepare the tofu.
5. Rinse it, pat it dry with absorbent paper, and then cut it into cubes.
6. Heat a spoonful of olive oil in a pan and as soon as it is hot, sauté the tofu for 3 minutes.

7. Peel and remove the seeds from the melon and then cut it into cubes.
8. Wash and dry the mint leaves.
9. As soon as 10 minutes have passed, take the couscous and season it with oil, salt and pepper.
10. Now put the olives, melon and tofu in the bowl with the couscous.
11. Season with oil, salt, pepper and lemon juice and mix.
12. Decorate with mint leaves and serve.

Veggies Couscous

PREPARATION TIME: 10 minutes

COOKING TIME: 15 minutes
CALORIES: 185

INGREDIENTS FOR 4 SERVINGS
- 160 grams of couscous
- 100 grams of cherry tomatoes
- 2 of zucchini
- 2 of eggplants
- 100 grams of peas
- 1 garlic clove
- 1 teaspoon of grated fresh ginger
- 1 teaspoon of turmeric
- Olive oil to taste
- Salt and pepper to taste

DIRECTIONS
1. Start with preparing the vegetables. Wash the cherry tomatoes and cut them into 4 wedges.
2. Wash the zucchini and cut them into rings.
3. Wash the eggplants and cut them into cubes.
4. Rinse the peas and then let them drain.
5. Peel and wash the garlic and then chop it.
6. Fry the garlic in a pan with a tablespoon of oil.

7. As soon as it is golden brown, add the eggplants first. Stir and cook for 3 minutes.
8. Then add the rest of the vegetables. Season with salt and pepper and mix well.
9. Add ginger and turmeric, a glass of water and cook for another 10 minutes.
10. Meanwhile, prepare the couscous.
11. Put the couscous in a bowl and cover it with 350 ml of boiling water.
12. Cover the bowl and let the couscous absorb all the water.
13. As soon as it is ready, season with oil, salt and pepper.
14. Now add the vegetables, mix well and then serve.

Rice recipes

Brown rice with pumpkin and sage

PREPARATION TIME: 15 minutes
COOKING TIME: 45 minutes
CALORIES: 350

INGREDIENTS FOR 4 SERVINGS
- 320 grams of brown rice
- 200 grams of pumpkin already peeled
- 2 shallots
- 1 litre of vegetable broth
- sage leaves
- A teaspoon of ground cinnamon
- 30 grams of soy butter
- Salt and pepper to taste

DIRECTIONS
1. Wash the pumpkin and then cut it into cubes.
2. Peel and wash the shallots and then chop them.
3. Put a tablespoon of oil in a saucepan and put the shallot to brown for a couple of minutes.
4. Add the cinnamon and mix.
5. Now add the pumpkin and leave it to flavour for 2 minutes, stirring often.
6. Now add the rice and toast it for 3 minutes.

7. Cover the rice with the vegetable broth and cook for 30 minutes, stirring often.
8. Meanwhile, wash and dry the sage leaves.
9. Put the butter in a pan and let it melt. Now add the sage and sauté for 5 minutes.
10. As soon as the rice is cooked, turn it off and put it on the plates.
11. Sprinkle it with the sage butter and serve.

Brown rice with walnuts

PREPARATION TIME: 10 minutes
COOKING TIME: 25 minutes
CALORIES: 412

INGREDIENTS FOR 4 SERVINGS
- 320 grams of brown rice
- 60 grams of shelled walnuts
- 1 onion
- Olive oil to taste
- Salt and pepper to taste
- Hot vegetable broth to taste

DIRECTIONS
1. Start with the walnuts. Take a non-stick pan and put the walnuts to toast for a couple of minutes. Turn off, let them cool and then chop them.
2. Peel and wash the onion, then chop it.
3. Take a pot with high sides, pour a drizzle of extra virgin olive oil and fry the onion over low heat.
4. Now add the rice and toast it for a couple of minutes, stirring constantly to keep it from burning.
5. Now add two ladles of vegetable broth and stir until the rice has completely absorbed the broth.

6. Continue with the same procedure until the rice is well cooked.
7. At this point, season with salt and pepper, stir one last time and then turn off.
8. Add the chopped walnuts and mix to incorporate them into the rice.
9. Put the rice on serving plates, season with a drizzle of oil and serve.

Cherry tomato curry and black rice

PREPARATION TIME: 20 minutes
COOKING TIME: 40 minutes

CALORIES: 522

INGREDIENTS FOR 4 SERVINGS
For the curry
- 1 shallot
- 20 grams of grated ginger
- 2 cloves of garlic
- 1 red pepper
- 1 teaspoon of turmeric
- 1 teaspoon of Garam masala
- 500 grams of cherry tomatoes
- 1 sprig of chopped parsley
- Olive oil to taste
- Salt and pepper to taste

For the rice
- 280 grams of black rice
- 60 grams of soy butter
- 1 teaspoon of cilantro
- Salt and pepper to taste

DIRECTIONS
1. Peel and wash the shallot and then cut it into slices.

2. Wash the cherry tomatoes and then cut them in half.
3. Wash the chilli and then cut it into slices.
4. Peel and wash the garlic, then cut it into slices.
5. Put two tablespoons of oil in a pan and as soon as it is hot, add the shallot, garlic, ginger and chilli. Sauté for 5 minutes, stirring constantly.
6. Now add the turmeric and Garam masala and cook for another minute.
7. Add the cherry tomatoes, season with salt and pepper and mix.
8. Also, add 150 ml of hot water and cook for 20 minutes, stirring often.
9. Now switch to rice. Melt the butter in a saucepan. As soon as it has melted, put the rice to toast for 2 minutes.
10. Add the coriander, salt, pepper, and mix.
11. Add the broth and cook for 40 minutes, stirring often.
12. After 40 minutes, put it in a bowl.
13. Add the cherry tomatoes, mix well and then put on plates and serve.

Brown rice with cherry tomatoes and vegan mozzarella

PREPARATION TIME: 20 minutes

COOKING TIME: 30 minutes
CALORIES: 283

INGREDIENTS FOR 4 SERVINGS
- 240 grams of brown rice
- 4 basil leaves
- 12 cherry tomatoes
- 1 plant based mozzarella
- 1 shallot
- Olive oil to taste
- Salt and pepper to taste

DIRECTIONS
1. Wash and dry the basil leaves.
2. Put them in a pot with plenty of water and salt and bring to a boil.
3. Meanwhile, wash the cherry tomatoes and cut them in half.
4. Cut the mozzarella into cubes.
5. Peel, wash and chop the shallot.
6. As soon as the water comes to a boil, add the rice and

cook for 25 minutes.
7. As soon as it is cooked, drain and set aside.
8. Put two tablespoons of olive oil in a pan and brown the shallot for 2 minutes.
9. Add the cherry tomatoes and sauté for 3 minutes.
10. Season with salt and pepper, mix and add the rice and mozzarella.
11. Stir, cook for a minute and then turn off.
12. Put the rice on the plates and serve.

Brown rice with spinach and raisins

PREPARATION TIME: 20 minutes
COOKING TIME: 30 minutes

CALORIES: 430

INGREDIENTS FOR 4 SERVINGS
- 320 grams of brown rice
- 300 grams of spinach
- A shallot
- 1 litre of vegetable broth
- 1 tablespoon of raisins
- 50 grams of soy butter
- Salt and pepper to taste

DIRECTIONS
1. Put the raisins to soften in a bowl with cold water.
2. Wash the spinach and let it drain and then chop it.
3. Peel and wash the shallot and then chop it.
4. Melt a little butter in a saucepan and then put the shallot to brown for a couple of minutes.
5. Stir and add the spinach and cook for 4 minutes, stirring often.
6. Now add the rice and toast it for 3 minutes, stirring constantly.

7. Season with salt and pepper and start adding the broth, one ladle at a time, stirring constantly. Remember that to add the other ladle the previous one must be completely absorbed.
8. Proceed in this way until the rice is cooked, about 25-30 minutes.
9. When the rice is cooked, squeeze the raisins and put them in the pot with the rice.
10. Continue to cook, for another 2 minutes.
11. Now put the butter and mix until it is completely absorbed.
12. Turn off, put the rice on the plates and serve.

Brown rice with spinach and raisins

PREPARATION TIME: 10 minutes
COOKING TIME: 35 minutes

CALORIES: 405

INGREDIENTS FOR 4 SERVINGS
- 320 grams of brown rice
- 2 bay leaves
- 4 carrots
- 1 tablespoon of curry
- Olive oil to taste
- Salt and pepper to taste

DIRECTIONS
1. Wash the bay leaves and put them in a pot with the rice. Cover with cold water and bring to a boil.
2. Now add the salt and pepper and continue cooking for another 20 minutes, covering the pot with a lid.
3. Meanwhile, peel the carrots, wash them and cut them into thin slices.
4. Heat two tablespoons of olive oil in a pan.
5. As soon as it is hot, put the carrots to sauté for 3 minutes.
6. Now add the curry and mix.

7. Cook for 5 minutes, then season with salt and pepper.
8. Now drain the rice and put it in the pan with the carrots. Stir and continue cooking for another 3 minutes.
9. Turn off, put the rice on the plates and serve.

Black rice with tofu, broad beans and cherry tomatoes

PREPARATION TIME: 20 minutes
COOKING TIME: 50 minutes

CALORIES: 568

INGREDIENTS FOR 4 SERVINGS
- 240 grams of black rice
- 300 grams of broad beans
- 200 grams of tofu
- 200 grams of cherry tomatoes
- 2 tablespoons of capers
- 1 clove of garlic
- 1 shallot
- 1 tablespoon of apple cider vinegar
- 1 teaspoon of mustard
- Olive oil to taste
- Salt and pepper to taste

DIRECTIONS
1. Wash the beans and let them drain.
2. Boil in water and salt and then cook the beans for a couple of minutes.
3. Drain them, pass them under cold and remove the skin

with a knife.
4. Wash the cherry tomatoes and cut them in half.
5. Put the cherry tomatoes in a bowl and season with 1 tablespoon of oil, salt and pepper. Mix and season well.
6. Bring a pot of water and salt to a boil and then put the rice to cook.
7. The rice will be cooked in about 40 minutes.
8. Meanwhile, pat the tofu with absorbent paper and then cut it into cubes.
9. Heat a pan with a little oil and sauté the tofu for 3 minutes.
10. As soon as it is cooked, season with salt and pepper and turn off.
11. As soon as it is cooked, drain it, put it in a bowl, and let it cool for 10 minutes.
12. Peel and wash the garlic and shallots and then chop them.
13. Put a tablespoon of oil in a pan and as soon as it is hot, brown the garlic and shallot.
14. After a couple of minutes, add the beans.
15. Cook for 5 minutes, season with salt and pepper and then transfer the beans to the bowl with the rice.
16. Now add the cherry tomatoes, tofu, and mix well.
17. In a small bowl, emulsify the apple cider vinegar,

mustard, oil, salt and pepper.

18. Pour the emulsion over the rice and mix everything well.

19. Put the rice on the plates and serve.

Vegetarian Buddha bowl

PREPARATION TIME: 20 minutes
COOKING TIME: 40 minutes

CALORIES: 360

INGREDIENTS FOR 4 SERVINGS
- 160 grams of black rice
- 4 carrots
- 1 broccoli
- 2 avocados
- Soy sauce to taste
- Salt and Pepper To Taste.
- Olive oil to taste

DIRECTIONS
1. Peel and wash the carrots and then cut them into strips.
2. Remove the broccoli flowers and then wash them and let them drain.
3. Put the broccoli flowers and carrots to steam for 15 minutes.
4. Meanwhile, put the rice to cook in salted boiling water for 40 minutes.
5. As soon as the rice is cooked, drain it and put it in a bowl.

6. Season it with oil, pepper, and mix.
7. Now peel the avocados, wash them, cut them in half and then remove the stone.
8. Now cut it into slices.
9. Now compose the bowls. Put the rice on the bottom, and then put the avocado slices, carrots and broccoli.
10. Drizzle with oil, sprinkle with soy sauce and serve.

Beetroot brown rice

PREPARATION TIME: 10 minutes
COOKING TIME: 40 minutes

CALORIES: 410

INGREDIENTS FOR 4 SERVINGS
- 320 grams of brown rice
- 40 grams of soy butter
- 2 small beets already cooked
- 800 ml of vegetable broth
- Salt and pepper to taste
- Olive oil to taste

DIRECTIONS
1. Start with the beets. Cut them into small pieces and put them in the glass of the blender. Blend them until you get a sort of puree.
2. Put a tablespoon of olive oil in a saucepan and put the rice to toast for a couple of minutes.
3. Add the vegetable broth and stir constantly.
4. As soon as the broth is completely consumed, add another ladle, always continuing to mix.
5. Proceed with this until the rice is cooked.
6. When cooked, add the beetroot purée and mix well.

7. Season with salt and pepper, stir again and then turn off.
8. Now add the butter cut into small pieces, and stir until the butter is completely incorporated.
9. Now put the rice on the plates and serve.

Brown rice with watermelon and tofu

PREPARATION TIME: 15 minutes
COOKING TIME: 40 minutes
CALORIES: 420

INGREDIENTS FOR 4 SERVINGS
- 500 grams of watermelon
- 320 grams of black rice
- 200 grams of grilled tofu
- 1 cucumber
- 2 limes
- 8 mint leaves
- Salt and Pepper to taste
- Olive oil to taste

DIRECTIONS
1. Start with preparing the rice. Bring the water and salt to a boil and then cook the rice for 35 minutes.
2. As soon as it is ready, drain it and place it in a bowl to cool.
3. Meanwhile, peel the watermelon and remove the seeds, then cut it into cubes.
4. Wash the cucumber and then cut it into slices.
5. Cut the tofu into cubes and put it in the bowl with the

rice.
6. Add the watermelon, cucumber, and mix.
7. Wash and dry the mint leaves and place them in the bowl.
8. Put the lime juice, a tablespoon of olive oil, salt and pepper in a small bowl and emulsify everything with a fork.
9. Season the rice with the emulsion, mix to flavour well and serve.

Black rice with pumpkin and pears

PREPARATION TIME: 20 minutes
COOKING TIME: 40 minutes

CALORIES: 388

INGREDIENTS FOR 4 SERVINGS
- 280 grams of black rice
- 350 grams of pumpkin
- 2 pears
- 3 zucchinis
- Half a shallot
- 1 litre of vegetable broth
- Olive oil to taste
- Salt and pepper to taste

DIRECTIONS
1. Wash the courgettes and then cut them into slices.
2. Peel the pears, wash and dry them. Cut them in half, remove the seeds and then cut them into cubes.
3. Peel and wash the shallot and then chop it.
4. Peel the pumpkin and remove the seeds. Wash the pulp and then cut it into cubes.
5. Put a tablespoon of oil in a saucepan and then put the shallot to brown for a couple of minutes.

6. Add the rice and sauté for 2 minutes, and then add the pumpkin.
7. Stir, season with salt and pepper and then add 2 ladles of broth.
8. Let the broth completely absorb, stirring constantly, and then add two more ladles of broth. Repeat the same operation until you have finished the broth.
9. 5 minutes before the end of cooking, add the pears and zucchinis.
10. Continue cooking for 5 minutes, stirring constantly and then turn off.
11. Put the rice on the plates, season with a drizzle of oil and serve.

Wholemeal risotto with saffron

PREPARATION TIME: 10 minutes
COOKING TIME: 35 minutes
CALORIES: 411

INGREDIENTS FOR 4 SERVINGS
- 320 grams of brown rice
- 1 onion
- 2 litres of vegetable broth
- 2 sachets of saffron
- 20 grams of soy butter
- 20 ml of olive oil
- Salt and pepper to taste

DIRECTIONS
1. Peel and wash the onion, then chop it.
2. Heat the oil in a saucepan and then put the onion to brown for a couple of minutes.
3. Now put the rice to toast for 3 minutes, stirring constantly.
4. Now pour a ladle of broth and let it absorb completely, always stirring.
5. Add another ladle and repeat the same previous operation.

6. Continue like this until the broth is completely used up.
7. Use the last ladle of broth to dissolve the saffron.
8. Pour it over the rice, mix and let it completely absorb.
9. Now add the butter, let it melt completely, always stirring and then turn off.
10. Put the rice on the plates and serve.

Brown rice with leeks, apples and curry

PREPARATION TIME: 25 minutes
COOKING TIME: 45 minutes

CALORIES: 245

INGREDIENTS FOR 4 SERVINGS
- 10 leeks
- 2 apples
- Half a lemon
- 1 tablespoon of curry
- 500 ml of coconut milk
- 320 grams of brown rice
- Olive oil to taste
- Salt and pepper to taste

DIRECTIONS
1. Remove the outer leaves of the leeks, wash them and then cut them into 8 pieces.
2. Put a tablespoon of olive oil in a pan and as soon as it is hot, brown the leeks.
3. Brown them for a couple of minutes, and then season with salt, pepper, and mix.
4. Now add the coconut milk and curry, put the lid on and cook over low heat until the leeks are soft.

5. Meanwhile, peel the apples, remove the seeds, wash them and then cut them into slices.
6. Put them in a bowl and sprinkle them with the lemon juice.
7. Let them rest for 10 minutes, then put them in a pan with a little oil and cook for 5 minutes.
8. As soon as the leeks are soft enough, add the rice and mix.
9. Add 600 ml of water and bring to a boil.
10. Stir and continue cooking for another 10 minutes.
11. As soon as it is cooked, season with salt and pepper and turn off.
12. Put the rice and leeks on serving plates, put the apples on top of the rice and their cooking juices and serve.

Brown rice with tomato and herbs

PREPARATION TIME: 20 minutes
COOKING TIME: 35 minutes

CALORIES: 466

INGREDIENTS FOR 4 SERVINGS
- 320 grams of brown rice
- 300 grams of tomato sauce
- 2 plant based mozzarella
- 1 litre of vegetable broth
- 1 shallot
- 1 teaspoon of paprika
- 1 teaspoon of thyme leaves
- 1 teaspoon of rosemary needles
- The grated rind of one lemon
- Olive oil to taste
- Salt and pepper to taste

DIRECTIONS
1. Peel and wash the shallot.
2. Put a tablespoon of oil in a saucepan and put the shallot to dry for a couple of minutes.
3. When it is transparent, add the rice and toast for a few minutes.

4. Add a ladle of vegetable broth, paprika and tomato sauce. Cook the risotto as usual, stirring often with a wooden spoon and adding a ladle of hot broth when the previous one is absorbed.
5. When cooked, season with salt and pepper and add the diced mozzarella, thyme, lemon zest and rosemary.
6. Stir to flavour well and turn off.
7. Put the rice on the plates and serve.

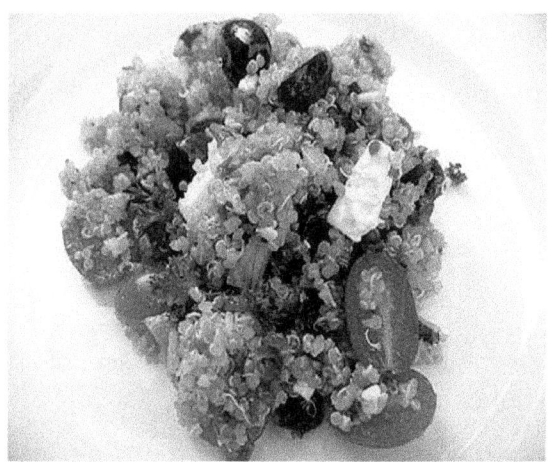

Black rice salad with mixed vegetables and pine nuts

PREPARATION TIME: 20 minutes

COOKING TIME: 25 minutes
CALORIES: 348

INGREDIENTS FOR 4 SERVINGS
- 280 grams of black rice
- 1 red pepper
- 1 yellow pepper
- 60 grams of mushrooms
- 1 shallot
- 1 lemon
- 30 grams of pine nuts
- 10 strands of chopped chives
- Salt and pepper to taste.
- Olive oil to taste

DIRECTIONS
1. Bring water and salt to a boil in a saucepan and cook the rice for 25 minutes.
2. Drain it and then put it in a bowl and let it cool.
3. Season with oil, salt, pepper, lemon juice, pine nuts and chives. Mix well.

4. Cut the peppers in half, remove the seeds and white filaments and then wash them. Cut them into strips.
5. Peel and wash the shallot and then cut it into slices.
6. Wash and dry the mushrooms and then cut them into slices.
7. Now put all the vegetables in the bowl with the rice.
8. Stir, to evenly distribute all the ingredients.
9. Divide the rice into serving plates and serve.

Brown rice with lentils

PREPARATION TIME: 20 minutes
COOKING TIME: 40 minutes
CALORIES: 301

INGREDIENTS FOR 4 SERVINGS
- 240 grams of brown rice
- 100 grams of lentils
- 1 carrot
- 2 shallots
- 1 sprig of rosemary
- 1 hot pepper
- 2 bay leaves
- Olive oil to taste
- Salt to taste

DIRECTIONS
1. Peel and wash the carrot and shallots, then chop them.
2. Wash and dry the bay leaves
3. Put the shallots, bay leaf and carrot in a pan with hot olive oil.
4. Fry for a couple of minutes and then add the lentils.
5. Sauté for a minute and then add 200 ml of water.

6. Cook the lentils for 30 minutes. Season with salt and pepper and turn off as soon as they are ready
7. In the meantime, prepare the rice.
8. Bring a pot of water and salt to a boil and then cook the rice for about 25 minutes. In any case, always follow the instructions on the package.
9. Just cooked, drain the rice and set it aside for a few minutes.
10. Wash and dry the rosemary and cut it into small pieces.
11. Put a tablespoon of olive oil in a pan and when it is hot, put the rosemary to fry.
12. Now add the rice and sauté for a minute and then add the lentils. Season with salt and pepper, stir and continue cooking for another minute and turn off.
13. Wash the red pepper and chop it, then put it in the pan with the rice.
14. Stir once more, then transfer the rice to serving plates and serve.

Black rice with peas cream

PREPARATION TIME: 20 minutes
COOKING TIME: 35 minutes

CALORIES: 377

INGREDIENTS FOR 4 SERVINGS
- 320 grams of black rice
- 250 grams of peas
- 1 shallot
- the grated zest of a lemon
- 100 ml of vegetable broth
- olive oil to taste
- salt and pepper to taste

DIRECTIONS
1. Peel and wash the shallot and then chop it.
2. Rinse the peas under running water and then let them drain.
3. Brown the shallot in a pan with a tablespoon of olive oil.
4. As soon as it is golden brown, add the peas.
5. Season with salt and pepper, mix and sauté for a couple of minutes.
6. Now add the vegetable broth and let them cook for 10

minutes.

7. After 10 minutes, add the lemon zest, mix and then blend everything with an immersion blender.
8. Now prepare the rice. Boil a pot with water and salt and then put the rice to cook following the instructions on the package.
9. As soon as it is cooked, drain it and put it in a bowl.
10. Add the pea cream and mix well.
11. Put the rice on serving plates and serve.

Soup recipes

Board beans cream

PREPARATION TIME: 15 minutes
COOKING TIME: 30 minutes
CALORIES: 72

INGREDIENTS FOR 4 SERVINGS
- 600 grams of fresh broad beans
- 800 ml of vegetable broth
- 1 shallot
- A tablespoon of cumin seeds
- Olive oil to taste
- Salt and pepper to taste

DIRECTIONS
1. Shell the beans, remove the skin and then wash them.
2. Peel and wash the shallot and then chop it.
3. Heat two tablespoons of olive oil in a saucepan.
4. As soon as it is hot, brown the shallot for a couple of minutes.
5. Add the broad beans and cumin and sauté them for 10 minutes, stirring often.

6. Now add the vegetable broth and continue cooking for another 15 minutes.
7. Lower the heat and blend everything with an immersion blender.
8. Continue cooking for another 2 minutes, stirring constantly.
9. Turn off, put the cream on the plates, season with olive oil and serve.

Peas cream

PREPARATION TIME: 15 minutes

COOKING TIME: 25 minutes
CALORIES: 60

INGREDIENTS FOR 4 SERVINGS

- 300 grams of peas
- 1 onion
- 5 mint leaves
- Salt and pepper to taste
- Olive oil to taste

DIRECTIONS
1. Peel and wash the onion then chop it.
2. Rinse the peas under running water and then let them drain.
3. Put a tablespoon of olive oil in a saucepan and as soon as it is hot, put the onion to fry for a couple of minutes.
4. Now add the peas, mix and season with salt and pepper.
5. Now add 300 ml of water and cook for 20 minutes.
6. After 20 minutes, take half of the peas and set them aside.
7. Blend the rest with an immersion blender until you get a smooth and creamy mixture.
8. Wash and dry the mint leaves and then chop them.
9. Put the whole peas back into the pot with the mint.
10. Stir, leave to flavor for 2 minutes and then turn off.

11. Put the cream on the plates, season it with a drizzle of olive oil and serve.

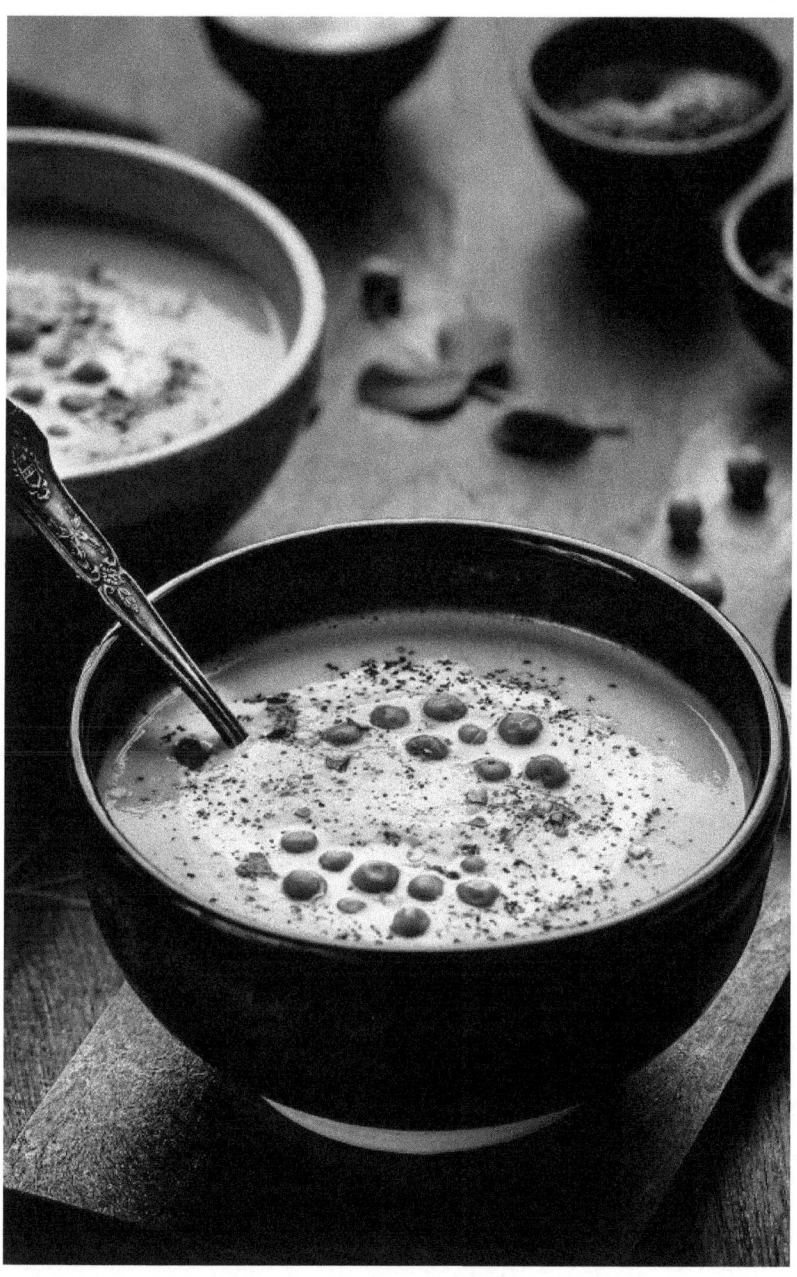

Lentils stewed with peppers and shallots

PREPARATION TIME: 15 minutes
COOKING TIME: 40 minutes

CALORIES: 304

INGREDIENTS FOR 4 SERVINGS
- 280 grams of lentils
- 2 yellow peppers
- 2 shallots
- 1 sprig of rosemary
- 2 teaspoons of turmeric
- 500 ml of vegetable broth
- Salt and Pepper To Taste.
- Olive oil to taste

DIRECTIONS
1. Peel and wash the shallots and then cut them into thin slices.
2. Remove the top cap from the peppers, cut them in half, remove the seeds and white filaments and then wash them. Cut them into slices that are not too large.
3. Heat a tablespoon of oil in a pan.
4. As soon as it is hot enough, add the shallots and brown them for a couple of minutes.

5. Now add the peppers, stir and cook for another 5 minutes.
6. Now add the lentils, mix, season with salt and pepper and then cover everything with the vegetable broth.
7. Cook for another 30 minutes, stirring often.
8. Meanwhile, wash and dry the rosemary and remove the needles.
9. After 30 minutes, add the rosemary needles and turmeric to the lentils and continue cooking for another 5 minutes.
10. Turn off, transfer to serving dishes, season with a drizzle of oil and serve.

Sweet potato soup

PREPARATION TIME: 20 minutes

COOKING TIME: 25 minutes
CALORIES: 313

INGREDIENTS FOR 4 SERVINGS
- 400 grams of sweet potatoes
- 100 grams of corn kernels
- 1 shallot
- 1 clove of garlic
- 80 ml of soy cream
- 2 litres of vegetable broth
- 1 teaspoon of thyme leaves
- Olive oil to taste
- Salt and pepper to taste

DIRECTIONS
1. Peel and wash the shallots and garlic and then chop them.
2. Peel the sweet potatoes, wash them and then dry them. Cut them into cubes.
3. Put a tablespoon of oil in a saucepan. As soon as it is hot, brown the garlic and shallot.
4. After 2 minutes, add the sweet potatoes and vegetable

broth.

5. Cook for 15 minutes.
6. Now add the corn and season with salt and pepper.
7. Cook for another 5 minutes and then add the cream.
8. Stir and then turn off.
9. Put the soup on the plates, sprinkle them with the thyme leaves and serve.

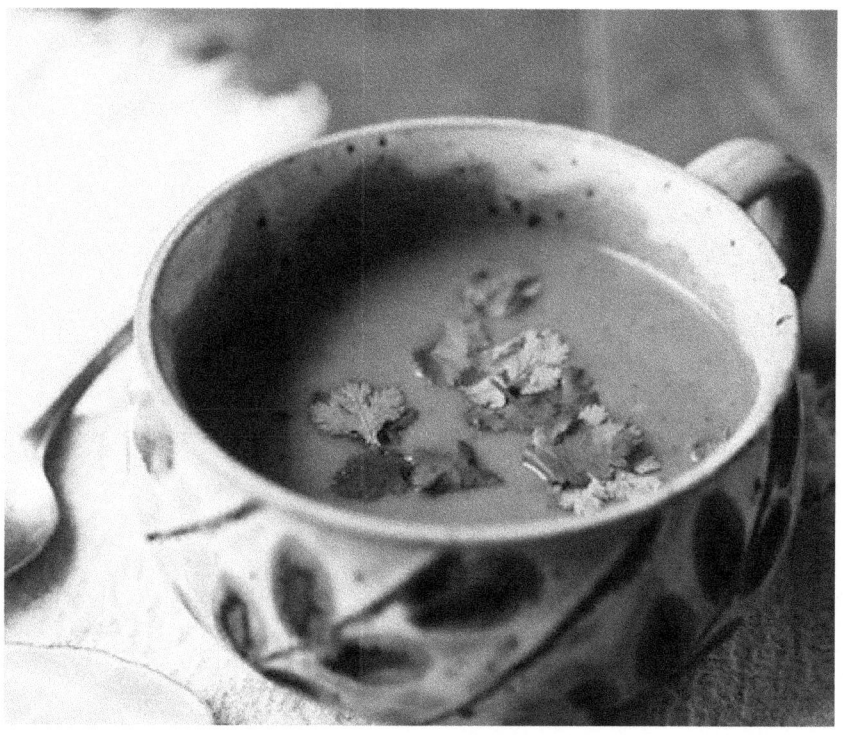

Bean and cabbage soup

PREPARATION TIME: 20 minutes
COOKING TIME: 2 hours

CALORIES: 240

INGREDIENTS FOR 4 SERVINGS

- 200 grams of cabbage leaves
- 150 grams of beans already soaked
- 1 carrot
- 1 shallot
- 100 grams of tomato pulp
- 4 bay leaves
- 2.5 litres of vegetable broth
- Olive oil to taste
- Salt and pepper to taste

DIRECTIONS
1. Put the broth in a saucepan and add the beans.
2. Bring to a boil and continue cooking for another 20 minutes.
3. Meanwhile, wash the cabbage leaves, dry them and cut them into strips.
4. Peel the carrot, wash it and then cut it into cubes.
5. Peel and wash the shallot and then chop it.

6. Wash and dry the bay leaves.
7. After 20 minutes, add the cabbage to the beans.
8. Stir and after 5 minutes add the carrot, shallot, bay leaves and tomato pulp.
9. Season with salt and pepper, stir and continue cooking for another 30 minutes.
10. After 30 minutes, turn off and remove the bay leaves.
11. Put the soup on plates, season with oil and pepper and serve.

Soup with red onion

PREPARATION TIME: 20 minutes
COOKING TIME: 40 minutes
CALORIES: 340

INGREDIENTS FOR 4 SERVINGS
- 200 grams of cabbage
- 2 carrots
- 1 potato
- 2 sticks of celery
- 1 red onion
- 100 grams of beans already boiled
- 100 grams of tomato pulp
- 2 litres of vegetable broth
- Salt and pepper to taste
- Olive oil to taste

DIRECTIONS
1. Wash and dry the cabbage leaves. Keep only the tenderest leaves and then cut them into strips.
2. Peel and wash the carrot and then cut it into cubes.
3. Peel the potato, wash it well under running water and then cut it into cubes.
4. Remove the celery stalk and the side filaments. Wash it

and chop it.
5. Peel the onion, wash it, and then slice it.
6. Put the vegetable broth in a saucepan and as soon as it starts to boil, add the potato, cabbage, carrots and celery.
7. Stir, cook for a couple of minutes and then add the tomato pulp.
8. Season with salt, pepper, and cook for 30 minutes.
9. Now add the beans, stir and continue cooking for another 10 minutes.
10. As soon as it is cooked, turn off and put the soup on serving plates.
11. Season with a drizzle of oil, sprinkle with onion and serve.

Basil soup

PREPARATION TIME: 15 minutes

CALORIES: 280

INGREDIENTS FOR 4 SERVINGS
- 2 carrots
- 1 onion
- 1 potato
- 2 litres of hot vegetable broth
- 8 basil leaves
- Olive oil to taste
- Salt and pepper to taste

DIRECTIONS
1. Peel and wash the carrots and then cut them into slices.
2. Peel and wash the potato and then cut it into cubes.
3. Peel and wash the onion and then cut it into thin slices.
4. Pour two tablespoons of olive oil into a saucepan and as soon as it is hot, add the onion.
5. Sauté for 2 minutes and then add the carrots and potato.
6. Season with salt and pepper, stir and then add the broth.
7. Cook with a lid on for 30 minutes over medium heat.

8. Meanwhile, wash and dry the basil leaves and then cut them into small pieces.
9. After the cooking time, turn off and put the soup on the plates.
10. Season with a drizzle of oil, sprinkle with basil and serve.

Cream of onions

PREPARATION TIME: 20 minutes
COOKING TIME: 30 minutes
CALORIES: 238

INGREDIENTS FOR 4 SERVINGS
- 400 grams of white onions
- 200 grams of potatoes
- 50 grams of oat flour
- 40 grams of soy butter
- 1 sprig of chopped parsley
- 1 tablespoon of chopped dill
- 1 tablespoon of chopped chives
- Olive oil to taste
- Salt and pepper to taste

DIRECTIONS
1. Peel the potatoes, wash them carefully under running water and then cut them into small pieces,
2. Peel and wash the onions and then slice them.
3. Put the butter in a saucepan and let it melt.
4. As soon as it melts, put the onions to brown for 5 minutes, stirring constantly.
5. Now add the potatoes, flour, and mix.

6. Season with salt and pepper and then pour in 1 litre of water.
7. Cook for 20 minutes and then lower the heat and blend everything with an immersion blender.
8. Continue cooking for another 3 minutes and then turn off.
9. Put the soup on plates and season with a drizzle of olive oil.
10. Sprinkle with the chopped herbs and serve.

Cold cream of peppers and tofu

PREPARATION TIME: 20 minutes
COOKING TIME: 23 minutes
CALORIES: 215

INGREDIENTS FOR 4 SERVINGS
- 2 red peppers
- 2 shallots
- 240 grams of tomato pulp
- 80 grams of tofu
- Olive oil to taste
- Salt and pepper to taste

DIRECTIONS
1. Cut the peppers in half, remove the seeds and white filaments and then wash them.
2. Cut them into slices.
3. Peel the shallots, wash and chop them.
4. Put a tablespoon of olive oil in a saucepan and then brown the shallots for a couple of minutes.
5. Add the tomato pulp and mix.
6. Continue cooking for a couple of minutes and then add the peppers.
7. Add 350 ml of water and cook for 20 minutes.

8. Meanwhile, rinse the tofu and pat it dry with absorbent paper.
9. Cut it into cubes and sauté it for 3 minutes in a pan with a tablespoon of olive oil.
10. Season with salt and pepper, turn off and set aside.
11. As soon as the peppers are cooked, turn off and blend everything with an immersion blender.
12. Put the cream into four bowls. Add the tofu and when they have cooled, put the soups in the fridge until ready to serve.

Potato and carrot soup

PREPARATION TIME: 20 minutes
COOKING TIME: 20 minutes

CALORIES: 265

INGREDIENTS FOR 4 SERVINGS
- 400 grams of potatoes
- 300 grams of carrots
- 1 onion
- 1.5 litres of vegetable broth
- 40 grams of soy butter
- 2 sprigs of chopped parsley
- Salt and pepper to taste

DIRECTIONS
1. Peel the potatoes, wash them and then cut them into cubes.
2. Peel and wash the carrots and then cut them into slices.
3. Peel and wash the onion and then chop it.
4. Put the vegetable broth in a saucepan and bring to a boil.
5. Put the carrots, potatoes, onion, and season with salt and pepper.
6. Cook for 20 minutes over medium heat.

7. After 20 minutes, turn off and blend everything with an immersion blender.
8. Put the butter cut into chunks and stir until melted.
9. Also, add the parsley and mix.
10. Now put the soup on the serving plates and serve.

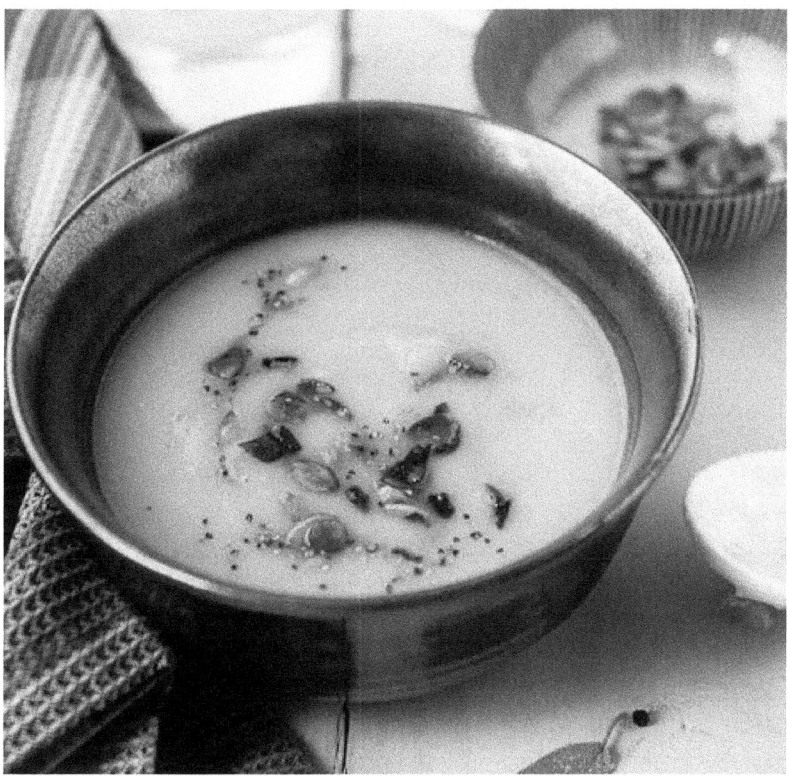

Chickpea, leek and rosemary soup

PREPARATION TIME: 15 minutes+2 hours to rest

COOKING TIME: 1 hour and 15 minutes
CALORIES: 225

INGREDIENTS FOR 4 SERVINGS
- 200 grams of chickpeas
- 3 leeks
- 2 sprigs of rosemary
- The grated rind of one lemon
- Olive oil to taste
- Salt and pepper to taste

DIRECTIONS
1. Start by putting the chickpeas in a bowl with cold water. Let it sit for 2 hours.
2. Remove the root and the green part of the leeks, wash them and then cut them into thin slices.
3. Put two tablespoons of oil in a saucepan and as soon as it is hot, put the leeks to dry.
4. Cook them for about 10 minutes and then add the chickpeas. Mix and season with salt and pepper.
5. Now add 1 litre of water and bring to a boil.
6. Wash the rosemary, and put it in the pot with the

chickpeas and continue cooking for another 60 minutes.
7. When cooked, remove the rosemary and take half of the soup.
8. Put it in the blender glass and blend until thick and creamy.
9. Put it back in the pot with the rest of the chickpeas and add the grated lemon zest.
10. Stir to flavour well. Put the soup on the plates and serve.

Spelt soup and porcini mushrooms

PREPARATION TIME: 15 minutes
COOKING TIME: 1 hour
CALORIES: 250

INGREDIENTS FOR 4 SERVINGS
- 200 grams of spelt
- 300 grams of porcini mushrooms
- 1 clove of garlic
- 1 shallot
- 1 sprig of chopped parsley
- Olive oil to taste
- Salt and pepper to taste

DIRECTIONS
1. Remove the earthy part of the mushrooms, wash them under running water and then dry them. Cut them into slices not too thin.
2. Peel and wash the shallot and then cut it into slices.
3. Peel and wash the garlic.
4. Put two tablespoons of oil in a saucepan and as soon as it is hot, brown the shallot and garlic.
5. As soon as they are golden brown, add the spelt and mix.

6. Sauté for a couple of minutes and then add the mushrooms.
7. Mix, season with salt and pepper and then add 1 litre of water.
8. Bring to a boil and then continue cooking over low heat for 40 minutes.
9. As soon as the soup is cooked, turn it off and put it on the plates.
10. Season with oil and chopped parsley and serve.

Zucchini and spinach soup

PREPARATION TIME: 10 minutes
COOKING TIME: 30 minutes
CALORIES: 110

INGREDIENTS FOR 4 SERVINGS
- 600 grams of zucchini
- 500 grams of spinach
- 2 tomatoes
- 1 carrot
- 1 onion
- 8 basil leaves
- Olive oil to taste
- Salt and pepper to taste

DIRECTIONS
1. Wash the zucchinis and then cut them into thin slices.
2. Wash and dry the spinach and then cut them into thin strips.
3. Peel and wash the onion and carrot and then chop them.
4. Wash and dry the basil leaves.
5. Wash the tomatoes and then cut them into cubes.
6. Pour a litre of water into a saucepan and put onion, carrots, tomatoes, spinach and zucchini inside.

7. Bring to a boil and season with salt and pepper.
8. Continue cooking for another 25 minutes.
9. After 25 minutes, drain some of the vegetables and put them in the glass of the blender together with the basil leaves. Blend until you get a smooth and homogeneous mixture.
10. Put the vegetable smoothie in the pot and bring to a boil again.
11. At this point, turn off, put the soup on the plates, season with a drizzle of oil and serve.

Lentil, oat and nut soup

PREPARATION TIME: 15 minutes

COOKING TIME: 1 hour and 15 minutes
CALORIES: 240

INGREDIENTS FOR 4 SERVINGS
- 250 grams of lentils
- 100 grams of tomato sauce
- 1 onion
- 1 carrot
- 2 tablespoons of cooked oats
- 20 nuts
- 2 bay leaves
- 1 clove of garlic
- Olive oil to taste
- Salt and pepper to taste

DIRECTIONS
1. Put the lentils in a bowl with cold water and let them rest for 2 hours.
2. Peel and wash the carrot, garlic and onion and then chop them.
3. Wash and dry the bay leaves.
4. Put a tablespoon of olive oil in a saucepan and as soon as it is hot, sauté the chopped vegetables and bay leaf.

5. Stir and after a couple of minutes add the tomato puree.
6. Mix well and add the lentils. Season with salt and pepper, stir, and add a liter of water.
7. Bring to a boil, then lower the heat and continue cooking for another hour.
8. Now remove the bay leaves and add the walnuts and oats.
9. Stir, cook for 2-3 minutes and then turn off.
10. Put the soup on the plates, season it with a drizzle of oil and serve.

Corn chowder

PREPARATION TIME: 15 minutes
COOKING TIME: 35 minutes
CALORIES: 238

INGREDIENTS FOR 4 SERVINGS
- 800 grams of corn already shelled
- 1 litre of vegetable broth
- 400 grams of potatoes
- 400 ml of soymilk
- 50 grams of soy butter
- 30 grams of corn starch
- 1 shallot
- 1 clove of garlic
- 1 teaspoon of paprika
- 1 sprig of chopped parsley
- Salt and pepper to taste

DIRECTIONS
1. Peel the potatoes, wash them and then cut them into cubes.
2. Rinse the corn kernels and then let them drain.
3. Peel and wash the shallot and garlic and then chop them.
4. Put the butter in a pan and let it melt.

5. Add the garlic and shallots and brown them for 1 minute.
6. Add the paprika and corn starch and mix. Cook for 30 seconds.
7. Now add the potatoes and the vegetable broth.
8. Cover and cook for 15 minutes.
9. Now add the corn kernels and continue cooking for another 15 minutes.
10. Stir, season with salt and pepper and turn off.
11. Take an immersion blender and blend everything by adding the milk a little at a time.
12. Blend until you have obtained a smooth and creamy mixture.
13. Put the soup on serving plates, season with a drizzle of oil and the chopped parsley and serve.

Lentil soup with cumin and lemon

PREPARATION TIME: 20 minutes
COOKING TIME: 1 hour and 10 minutes

CALORIES: 358

INGREDIENTS FOR 4 SERVINGS
- 400 grams of lentils
- 1 teaspoon of cumin seeds
- 1.5 litres of vegetable broth
- 1 lemon
- 1 shallot
- 1 carrot
- 1 bay leaf
- Salt and pepper to taste
- Olive oil to taste

DIRECTIONS
1. Peel and wash the carrot and shallot, then cut them into pieces.
2. Wash and dry the lemon and remove the zest.
3. Put carrot, onion and lemon zest in the mixer and chop.
4. Wash and dry the bay leaf.
5. Put 2 tablespoons of olive oil in a saucepan and heat it up.
6. Add the bay leaf and cumin seeds and sauté for a

minute.
7. Now add the chopped vegetables and mix.
8. As soon as the vegetables become soft, add the lentils.
9. Stir, season with salt and pepper and add the broth.
10. Cover the pot and cook for 1 hour over medium heat.
11. Stir occasionally and as soon as the lentils are ready, turn off.
12. Put the soup on the plates, season it with oil and serve.

Carrot cream and black rice

PREPARATION TIME: 20 minutes
COOKING TIME: 30 minutes
CALORIES: 150

INGREDIENTS FOR 4 SERVINGS
- 800 grams of carrots
- 2 potatoes
- 150 grams of black rice
- 1 lemon
- 5 chopped chives
- 1 litre of vegetable broth
- Olive oil to taste
- Salt and pepper to taste

DIRECTIONS
1. Peel and wash the carrots and then cut them into small pieces.
2. Peel and wash the potatoes thoroughly and then cut them into cubes.
3. Wash and dry the lemon. Cut it in half. Grate the zest of half a lemon. Peel the other half of the lemon and cut the pulp into cubes.
4. Bring the vegetable broth to a boil and then cook the potatoes and carrots.

5. Cook for 20 minutes, season with salt and pepper and then add the lemon zest.
6. While the vegetables are cooking, prepare the rice. Put the rice to boil in a pot with boiling water and salt following the cooking times shown in the box.
7. As soon as it is cooked, drain it and put it in a bowl. Season with the lemon pulp, oil, chopped chives and pepper. Stir to flavour the rice well.
8. As soon as the vegetables are cooked, turn off and blend everything with an immersion blender.
9. Put the soup on serving plates, arrange the rice in the centre, season with a drizzle of oil and serve.

Quinoa and spinach soup

PREPARATION TIME: 30 minutes
COOKING TIME: 50 minutes
CALORIES: 330

INGREDIENTS FOR 4 SERVINGS
- 150 grams of quinoa
- 8 mushrooms
- 1 clove of garlic
- 100 grams of spinach
- 2 litres of vegetable broth
- 2 teaspoons of grated ginger
- 1 onion
- 1 carrot
- 150 grams of tofu
- Salt and pepper to taste.
- Olive oil to taste

DIRECTIONS
1. Wash and dry the mushrooms and then cut them into slices.
2. Bring the vegetable broth to a boil and then add the mushrooms and ginger.
3. Cook for 20 minutes and then remove the mushrooms and turn off.

4. Peel the onion and carrots and then chop them.
5. Wash the spinach thoroughly and then pat dry.
6. Heat a tablespoon of olive oil in a saucepan and then put the onion and carrots to fry for 10 minutes.
7. Now add the vegetable broth and when it starts to boil, add the quinoa.
8. Cook over medium heat for 20 minutes.
9. When the quinoa is cooked, add the spinach, season with salt and pepper and mix well.
10. Turn off and let it sit for a couple of minutes.
11. Meanwhile, pat the tofu with absorbent paper and then cut it into cubes.

Lentil and broccoli soup

PREPARATION TIME: 30 minutes
COOKING TIME: 40 minutes

CALORIES: 154

INGREDIENTS FOR 4 SERVINGS
- 250 grams of lentils
- 200 grams of broccoli flowers
- 5 cherry tomatoes
- 1 carrot
- 1 shallot
- 500 ml of vegetable broth
- Olive oil to taste
- Salt and Pepper to taste

DIRECTIONS
1. Put the lentils in a bowl with water and let them rest overnight.
2. Wash and dry the broccoli flowers.
3. Peel and wash the carrot and shallot and then chop them.
4. Wash the cherry tomatoes and cut them in half.
5. Put a tablespoon of olive oil in a saucepan and when it

is hot, sauté the carrot and shallot for a couple of minutes.
6. Now add the cherry tomatoes, mix and sauté them for 3 minutes, then add the vegetable broth and lentils.
7. Cook for 20 minutes and then add the broccoli.
8. Continue cooking for another 15 minutes, season with salt, pepper, and turn off.
9. Put the soup on serving plates, drizzle with olive oil and serve.

Cream of tomato soup

PREPARATION TIME: 10 minutes

COOKING TIME: 20
CALORIES: 116

INGREDIENTS FOR 4 SERVINGS
- 600 grams of red tomatoes
- 1 red onion
- 4 slices of wholemeal bread
- 1 clove of garlic
- 10 stalks of chives
- Olive oil to taste
- Sale to taste
- Chilli powder to taste

DIRECTIONS
1. Wash and dry the tomatoes.
2. Bring some water to a boil and then blanch the tomatoes for 1 minute.
3. Drain them, let them cool by passing them under cold water and then remove the peel.
4. Cut them into cubes, eliminating the seeds and the vegetation water.
5. Peel and wash the onion and then cut it into thin slices.

6. Wash the chives and then chop it.
7. Heat a tablespoon of oil in a saucepan. As soon as it is hot, brown the onion for a couple of minutes.
8. Add the tomato. Season with salt and add the chilli and mix.
9. Cook for 10 minutes, stirring occasionally.
10. Add the chives and cook for another 5 minutes.
11. Meanwhile, prepare the bread.
12. Peel the garlic and wash it. Rub it on the slices of bread.
13. Put the bread to toast in the toaster, until it is crunchy enough.
14. As soon as the tomatoes are cooked, turn off and blend everything with an immersion blender.
15. Serve the cream in four individual bowls, season with a drizzle of oil, add the croutons and serve.

Carrot, pumpkin and black rice soup

PREPARATION TIME: 20 minutes
COOKING TIME: 50 minutes

CALORIES: 190

INGREDIENTS FOR 4 SERVINGS
- 400 grams of pumpkin pulp
- 120 grams of black rice
- 500 ml of vegetable broth
- 2 carrots
- 1 leek
- A pinch of nutmeg
- Olive oil to taste
- Salt and Pepper To Taste.

DIRECTIONS
1. Wash the pumpkin pulp and then cut it into cubes.
2. Wash the leek and cut it into thin slices.
3. Peel and wash the carrots and then cut into slices.
4. Heat a spoonful of olive oil in a saucepan and then brown the leek for a couple of minutes.
5. Add the pumpkin, mix and sauté for a minute.
6. Now add the vegetable broth, put the lid on and cook for 15 minutes.

7. Now add the carrots and cook for another 15 minutes, stirring occasionally.
8. After 15 minutes, add the rice. Season with salt, pepper, and mix.
9. Cook until the rice is al dente. At this point, add the nutmeg.
10. Stir one last time and then turn off.
11. Put the soup on the plates, season with a drizzle of oil and serve.

Lightning Source UK Ltd.
Milton Keynes UK
UKHW020651170621
385673UK00010B/711